d,
d

Praise

"This short but informative memoir, which features family photographs, showcases the author's straightforward voice and copious self-awareness...An illuminating look at the impact of a life-changing diagnosis."

–Kirkus Reviews

"Jim's book is a moving and heartfelt account of his life post-injury. He delves into the hard work and struggles of recovery, as well as his adaptation to a new and challenging lifestyle. Having known Jim for twenty-five years, I knew that he would persevere and make the best of an extremely difficult situation. However, his book gave me a real sense of what he and Mary have been through. His accomplishments after the injury are truly inspiring!"

—David B. Kynor, lecturer at the Thayer School of Engineering, Dartmouth College

"*Cracked* chronicles Jim Barry's story of survival following a traumatic brain injury. This detailed account takes the reader through the experience of the accident, rehab, and day-to-day life now, years after. It gives the reader an opportunity to look behind the first impression of disability. Jim's investment in this new life, very different from his past, speaks to his resilience, tenacity, and commitment to leading a good life."

—Jill Gravink, director, Northeast Passage

"*Cracked* is a no-nonsense story of a single-minde[d] tenacious man surviving a life-altering experience an[d] eventually thriving again, thanks to the help of his wife[,] family, and health professionals. I have known Jim for over forty years. His bicycle accident was a shock to many of us, and we wished him well from a distance. But we never fully appreciated the extraordinary struggles he went through for rehabilitation, both physical and mental. This book is a captivating testimony to his focused effort to move forward. It serves as an inspiration to us all on how never to give up."

—Michael L. Corradini, Wisconsin distinguished professor

"The journey of Jim Barry's *Cracked* is heartbreaking as well as heart lifting. It is hard to believe the trauma he endured, with its minute details that puts the reader in the thick of it. He kept track of his suffering with a spreadsheet (he is an engineer after all!) which informed the book's emotional backbone. He is quite funny in the telling although the reader can see the misery behind the mask. It is a story like no other. We can follow the emotional traces of our own injuries from the tracks of Jim's trail."

–Thomas G. Broussard, Jr., PhD, president & founder of Aphasia Nation, Inc.

"An engineer's insight into how to navigate a life-changing incident."

–Avery Demond, PhD

"*Cracked* gives the audience insight into the life of author Jim Barry after a mountain biking accident in the Northeast Kingdom of Vermont Through his lens, Jim recounts the moments leading up to the accident, first discovering the extent of his injuries, and the long road ahead as he navigates life's new challenges living with a traumatic brain injury. Jim's ability to clearly articulate a mixture of frustration, gratitude, disappointment, and finding the silver linings is an impressive illustration of what day-to-day life is like for him. Through his perseverance and the support of his family, Jim shifts the common narrative of disability, proving to the reader that he is still able to access a very full and adventurous life."

–Carly Bascom (she/her/hers), executive director of New England Healing Sports Association

"*Cracked* is an inspirational journey of resilience and moving forward in spite of the physical and mental uncertainties ahead after a severe traumatic brain injury. Jim's writing is insightful and in some ways therapeutic, while filled with a renewed self-awareness after the injury. The sharing of his experiences through this book may support others to thrive when confronted with similar life-changing circumstances."

–Camilo E. Fadul, MD, professor of neurology at University of Virginia

CRACKED

CRACKED

My Life After a Skull Fracture

Jim Barry

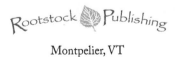

Rootstock Publishing

Montpelier, VT

First Printing: January 2023

Cracked, Copyright © 2022 by Jim Barry

All Rights Reserved.

Release Date: 01/31/23

Softcover ISBN: 978-1-57869-122-7
Hardcover ISBN: 978-1-57869-123-4
eBook ISBN: 978-1-57869-124-1

Library of Congress Control Number: 20229158534

Published by Rootstock Publishing
an imprint of Multicultural Media, Inc.
27 Main Street, Suite 6
Montpelier, VT 05602 USA

www.rootstockpublishing.com

info@rootstockpublishing.com

Interior and cover design by Eddie Vincent, ENC Graphic Services (ed.vincent@encirclepub.com)

Author photo by Courtney Cania

For permissions or to schedule an author interview, contact the author at jimbarry2001@gmail.com

Printed in the USA

Preface

"If you don't stop that, you'll fall and break your skull."
That's what my mom used to say when I was a kid. Of course, Mom was right. Though it took a lot of years, I did break my skull.

If you're reading this, I imagine it's because you or someone you love has had a traumatic brain injury (TBI), and you're trying to learn as much as you can about it. Let me state at the outset that brain injuries vary widely and that my story is representative only of me. I hope by sharing these thoughts and experiences that it may help someone cope with their own challenges, but I don't pretend that what I say is somehow universal.

With that out of the way, I suppose you're wondering exactly what happened. I broke my skull in a mountain biking crash (yes, I was wearing a helmet) with a subsequent cerebral hemorrhage. (In other words, I suffered a hemorrhagic stroke rather than the more common ischemic stroke: my brain was starved of blood flow by a leak rather than a blockage.) I broke a few ribs and a collarbone, too, but they healed. The fracture in my skull healed as well (with a big dent), but my brain was permanently altered.

I was never much of a daredevil. Prudent perhaps best describes me, though I have always nudged the limit of my fears. I guess I nudged once too often. So the broken skull is and isn't my own fault.

The injury occurred in the area of my brain stem. I lost my balance function along with most of my hearing. My right cornea was damaged irretrievably, and my left eye has a persistent nystagmus (twitch), so my sight is limited. Below the neck, I have extensive weakness and numbness on my left side. Since some key cranial nerves were disrupted, my face droops on the right. I get around mostly by wheelchair.

I try not to use medical jargon in this book, but two words are worth remembering: aphasia and neuroplasticity. Neither was ever spoken to me by medical staff, though I'm sure they were quite cognizant of those terms. Aphasia refers to the loss of communication that often occurs with brain injuries. It is a common outcome of stroke. Neuroplasticity is the ability of your brain to repurpose regions to restore functions. Though imperfect, it forms the basis of recovery from brain injuries.

The bright side of getting injured—there is a bright side?—is the amazing range of supportive people I met. While many were just doing their job, the way in which they cared for me felt inspiring. Organizations dedicated to helping disabled people were out there waiting to serve me. Family, friends, and colleagues also helped me along the way.

None of this means that becoming disabled is a net positive experience. All of us hope to not need the available services. Despite my frequent attempts at levity, I have had plenty of days when I wished for balance and moments when I can't accurately hear important words. I miss things and activities I gave up. Despair overwhelms me at times. The only answer I've found is to keep plowing forward and keep looking ahead. In fact, though a short introduction such as this is called a preface or, sometimes, a foreword,

I think the term *forward* would be more appropriate here.

The first five chapters of this book are largely chronological and detail the first eighteen months or so. The remainder of the chapters are grouped by topic since they all run together in time.

Part 1

The Initial Eighteen-Plus Months

Chapter 1

Prelude

"I have never seen someone last two years in their current situation with happiness numbers this low."

I had just taken one of those surveys that purports to assess your personality, and our employee assistance program (EAP) counselor had just scored it and now reported the results to me in private in a conference room. The EAP was a benefit to employees, provided by an outside firm. As president of the company, I had put myself forward as a trial of this new tool.

Why shouldn't I be happy? Was I just whining about the everyday things we all face? (I hate whining, especially when it comes from me.)

I was fifty-one years old, the president of the company for about six years. I had worked at the engineering research and development firm for over twenty years after earning my PhD from a top department in its field. The company had been extremely successful over the years and generally was regarded as a top player among smaller outfits. (We had roughly 130 employees.) The firm stood on stable ground.

I had a wonderful wife, a great son who was just entering his senior year in college, and two step-kids who were also well-launched. We had a beautiful home in an upscale New England college town plus a vacation home we'd built on a nearby lake, both paid for. I had (or could afford) all the toys I could want. I served as chair of a committee at my old university. The litany of great things could go on.

Just to complete the picture of bliss, I drove a four-wheel-drive crew-cab midsize pickup. It made it easy to tow the boats (we had a bunch) to and from the lake and haul bicycles (my passion) for various adventures. I was debating buying a convertible sports car (hello midlife crisis) and had even thought about a motorcycle. (It's ironic given what happened that I worried about hurting myself on a motorcycle.)

Still, the survey numbers were what they were, and I knew they had a point. I felt unsatisfied. Yet I knew how much I had going for me, and I was trying to hold on for a few more years. I believed that somehow everything would work itself out when I retired. Though retirement would come at an early age for me, I had no worries about being bored. I had lots of hobbies that would keep me busy.

Maybe I was just restless, I thought. Maybe I needed some sort of new challenge. No fundamental changes were needed to an already great life, I told myself.

I magically envisioned a retired life that would solve all my problems. I would live mostly out at the lake with lots of fishing and swimming and other watersports. I already served on the board of the lake association. As many retired folks do, my wife and I would get to travel. (My wife is a Europhile.) I had begun woodworking and had several new projects in mind. I intended to do some long bicycle tours. I was lucky that my wife also liked these trips. We had just wrapped a great cycling vacation in Northern Ireland, and I had always planned on a coast-to-coast bike tour of the US.

So I went on with life late that summer and early fall looking to make no changes. Aside from a bad fall waterskiing—I was never very good—the time passed. In September, we began a remodeling project on the master bath of the house in town and moved out to the lake.

In early October, I pulled the boats out of the water for the winter. The powerboat would go in for its end-of-season tune-up and get put away for the winter. I towed it down to the storage facility in my truck. The bigger sailboat would live on a trailer in our second garage at the house in town. The small sailboat, pedal boat, canoe, and kayaks could hang outside at the cottage on a rack I had built for a little longer before I hauled them indoors to the cottage basement for the winter. Pulling the boats out of the water always made me sad, but I had my weekends planned out, and it was time.

Despite being an avid winter sports enthusiast—with snow shoeing and both alpine and nordic skiing—I lived for the warm weather, so the end to the late spring/summer/ early fall season cast a pall. In addition to fishing and swimming, I sailed, snorkeled, and (poorly) water-skied. I loved the lake. Looking ahead, a positive thing for me about the cooler seasons was that I could spend the next few weeks in the woods without bugs. I hunted, but not very seriously, sort of just enough to maintain the tradition.

At work, the middle of fall meant prepping for the end of the fiscal year in December and the tricky setting of targets for corporate pay adjustment for the next year. I had done this all before, but it was never an easy process. Both activities required looking ahead into the coming year and foreseeing future circumstances.

The firm had successfully navigated a reauthorization of small business programs in the federal government (the company depended on these), which had entailed a few trips on my part to Washington to meet our elected representatives. With the reauthorization completed, the next few years had the potential to be healthy for the business.

I walked out of work that October Friday knowing that things would fall into place. (Maybe "fall" is a bad word choice.)

Chapter 2

Crash

"See ya Monday."

I probably said something like that as I walked out of the office on Friday. Little did any of us know that I wouldn't return for many Mondays to come.

It's funny to think about now, but my big debate on Saturday morning, October 12, 2012, was whether to stop for food somewhere.

The drive north from our home in Hanover, New Hampshire, to the mountain bike trail network at Kingdom Trails in the Northeast Kingdom of Vermont ran about an hour and a half. Foliage was just past peak, and the scenery looked beautiful. Leaving midmorning to let the day warm up a little meant that I arrived at the trails just before noon.

I had a peanut-butter sandwich and some energy bars in my hydration pack for later, but I was already feeling hungry, not an uncommon feeling for me. I forget what I had for breakfast that day, but the meal happened early and by late morning on the drive up I was ready for more food.

In those days I weighed close to 180 pounds. At about five foot ten, I was not overweight and was in good shape (I worked out frequently), but I had to pay close attention to what I ate. I was one of those people who had to eat frequently to maintain my blood sugar, so it was a delicate balancing act: eat enough to stave off the blood sugar fall but not enough to gain weight.

I ended up skipping the drive-thru that morning that I passed on the way to the trails. I had decided to get a few miles on the bike, then stop for something from my pack. I felt more virtuous that way. Little did I know that I wouldn't eat solid food for a year.

I stopped my truck as normal in the unpaved parking area at Kingdom Trails and began gearing up to ride. Another vehicle was nearby, and the occupants (two couples) were doing the same thing, talking in French. The trails were a popular place with the Quebecois (Canada was not far away), and it was not unusual to hear people conversing with each other in French. Despite four years of high school French and a wife who was fluent, I could only make out a few words.

It was late in the season, so the parking lot remained uncrowded. The temperature might have discouraged some people, since the day was only supposed to reach the high forties Fahrenheit, but it was sunny with no precipitation, so I was looking forward to the ride.

In addition to my hydration pack, I strapped on my helmet and installed the clear lenses in my cycling glasses. I wore leg warmers with my lycra cycling shorts and a yellow windbreaker over a synthetic tee and 100-weight synthetic pullover with lightweight gloves, fairly normal attire for the season. My bike was a full-suspension 29er that I had bought as a fiftieth birthday present about eighteen months before. Though just a medium, it was a big machine. The mountain bike dwarfed my usual road ride, a 57-centimeter frame.

I had ridden the 29er at Kingdom Trails several times in the past two cycling seasons. I loved the quality and variety of the trails. The big wheels of the bike and suspension let me roll over most trail surfaces with ease.

I didn't stop in the Kingdom Trails office that morning since I had a season pass for the trails, so I started biking on the paved road up Darling Hill. I was primarily a road cyclist, and this short uphill stretch on asphalt helped me warm up on the mountain bike. At the top of the hill the trails began with a series of green (beginner) routes that would help me adjust to the feel of off-road riding.

The ascent up the paved road felt normal (always steeper than I remembered from the last time). When I started off-road on the green trails at the top of the hill, something didn't feel right. It always took me a while to get into the rhythm of riding on dirt, so I wasn't seriously concerned.

When I hit a short rooty section of trail that I usually cleaned (if slowly), I had to stop and put a foot down. I was definitely not having a good day. I got through the roots and kept riding.

At the fork with the Tap'n'Die trail—a black diamond (expert) descent I had done a few times—I halted for a moment again. Tap'n'Die wound down the back side of the hill. At the bottom were some trails along a river where I often stopped to eat. That was my target again. I heard the elated cries of another group on the trail echoing through the forest. I started down.

The beginning of Tap'n'Die is easy. The trail doesn't achieve its black diamond status until further down. I had ridden it at least twice before, including once with my son, who was riding an old hardtail.

I did not feel confident. I navigated the upper section OK, though too slowly and tentatively. I pulled off the trail a couple times to let faster riders go by.

When I alpine skied, sometimes I started a day too uncertain as well. I often took myself to steeper terrain so that I would stop thinking and start reacting. I would push myself to get into the zone, to just begin to flow. After linking a few turns on steeper terrain when skiing, I usually relaxed and got the rhythm. I tried to do something similar on the mountain bike that day.

Near the bottom of Tap'n'Die, there are some short steep descents followed by short steep ascents, kind of like a roller coaster. I started to let the bike go more on the descents (less braking), to get more speed so I could roll up the mini-ascents with little pedaling.

On one of these roller coaster dips near the bottom of the trail not far from the river, I crashed.

I don't know exactly what happened. There were lots of fallen leaves, so I could have hit something that stopped my front wheel. A hidden rock? The fallen leaves certainly could have obscured it. Did I jam on the front brake when I sensed a problem? On a road bike, one is supposed to pull the front brake harder than the rear due to the weight shift. I have overdone braking off-road before, and the hydraulic brakes on my mountain bike grabbed very firmly. I had been using the rear brake to modulate my speed, though I could have reverted to road instincts and grabbed both brake levers hard in an emergency. A combination of things? I really don't know (as if it matters). I remember sailing through the air over the handlebars, then hitting the ground hard.

I never lost consciousness. I knew I had hit hard, but I expected to bounce up. I have wrecked off-road before and emerged essentially unscathed. I always used to say that it hadn't been a real mountain bike ride without shedding a little blood, though that was usually the result of riding through brambles.

But this time was different. I tried to reach my cycling glasses, which had fallen a few feet away, but I couldn't. My left hand shook and wouldn't work. Riders from a group appeared. I felt embarrassed to have crashed with others nearby. I tried to yell, but nothing would come out. I wanted to apologize to the other riders for interrupting their outing. Weekends were too short and precious to waste. Nothing. I showed the identification band on my left wrist by pointing to it with my right hand. More shaking.

Someone went up the hill for help (or at least far enough to get cell service). I just lay there on the cold ground on my back and waited, unable to move.

The first responders eventually came. As expected, they strapped me to a backboard due to concerns about my spine. They manually carried me out a short distance to a main trail along the river, then placed the backboard on a four-wheeler for the trip up the hill and out of the woods.

I remained conscious the whole time with no perceptible pain. My understanding now is that staying conscious and remembering are unusual with brain injuries.

Strapped to the backboard on the rear of the four-wheeler, I stared straight up and saw the blue sky. I mentally visualized the trails rescuers took up the hill. (I had ridden these trails on a prior visit.) The engine of the four-wheeler labored up the steep climb. Eventually the first-responders put me in an ambulance, I think at a farm on Darling Hill Road.

The ambulance pulled out and started heading to the hospital. I didn't know where a medical facility was, probably in Lyndonville. I felt them starting to cut away my jacket.

At some point in the ambulance ride, I began to lose consciousness. And I stopped breathing on my own. The attendants were apparently ready for that. I recall a mental image of little oxygen receptors slowly winking out. As the breathing mask was placed on my face, I remember making a deliberate decision to accept the air and wake up the receptors. Maybe I didn't have a choice, and it wasn't really my call, but it felt that way.

I recall thinking that this experience of being in a serious wreck would be interesting. I could stop it by refusing air (at least I thought I could), but it was more interesting to let it play out. Whether it was really my decision or not, it was the last time I felt some measure of free will for months.

I vaguely recall being rushed into a hospital, but that completes all my memories of the immediate aftermath.

My wife had worried when I had been gone too long, then she received one of those phone calls one hopes never to get. This call came from a hospital in Vermont. She rushed out and jumped in the car. She got only a few blocks away when she realized she didn't know where she was going, so she retreated home and called Dartmouth-Hitchcock Medical Center (DHMC)—a large teaching hospital only a couple miles from our home—to get directions.

The person at DHMC seemed happy to give her directions but told her that I had just been brought in by helicopter, so my wife's trek shrank to only a couple miles. Of course, I remember none of this.

My only other memory of that day is partially awaking inside a small chamber with flashing lights overhead. I have always assumed this chamber belonged to an MRI machine, though I suppose it might have been the helicopter.

Chapter 3

Hospitals

Previously when I visited hospitals, it had been in a white coat, not a patient johnny. In my career in R&D, I had sometimes seen doctors we collaborated with in clinical settings—some of my projects were biomedical—but I hadn't imagined myself in a hospital until I grew old and infirm.

Some Hospital in the Northeast Kingdom

I have no memories beyond getting rushed into the hospital to which I first arrived. In retrospect, I am guessing that it was Northern Vermont Regional Hospital, just north of St. Johnsbury. I am thankful to the people there, whatever the institution, for stabilizing me for transport.

Dartmouth-Hitchcock Medical Center

I don't remember being airlifted. To me, I suddenly awoke in a hospital. The idea of being in a medical facility didn't surprise me, since I knew I had been in a serious accident.

My memory of my stay at DHMC (just a couple miles

from my home in Hanover) remains quite spotty. I spent a couple weeks in the intensive care unit (ICU). Most of the time I was heavily sedated.

I remember partially waking and finding a spare arm in the bed. It must have been my left arm, which initially seemed disconnected. I remember some therapists giving me a computer, which I thought I could use but ended up staring at blankly. (The computer was a Mac and I was accustomed to PCs, but I doubt I could have made any sense of my own laptop.)

I remember waking briefly while undergoing a tracheostomy to help me breathe on my own. Not painful, but slightly disconcerting.

I remember some vivid dreams. What was left of my poor brain must have been trying to fashion a story from its strange inputs. I dreamed I was at work and somewhere in my truck, then I was out at the lake. I couldn't determine reality from a dream. Only in retrospect did I learn that I had (not surprisingly) never gone anywhere. I don't know if I had been placed on any meds that would help drive the dreams, though that fact wouldn't surprise me. To this day those dreams stay memorable though nonsensical.

I transitioned out of the ICU at some point, though saying I was spacey would be charitable. I had a vague sense of others discussing where I should go next, so some of my dreams focused on what I imagined rehab to be like. I vaguely recall some of the nursing staff, getting sponge baths, having lots of X-rays (the concern initially was my spine, which turned out to be fine), and being winched out of bed on a hoist and sitting on some sort of large object to begin my rehab.

During that period, my brother (a primary-care physician) had come from Tucson, and my son interrupted his senior year in college to hurry home. My wife spent long hours watching over me. As my brother remarked, I didn't have a mark on me, yet I was very seriously injured.

I can only imagine the scene occurring at the office, a combination of subdued, hopeful, and frantic all at once. Though things I did there posed no great mystery, my abrupt and unexpected absence could not have been easy. My wife delivered my laptop to help them navigate my sudden disappearance, but since key files were password-protected, I don't know how much it helped.

Several of my engineering colleagues came to visit me. I probably acknowledged them at the time, though I don't remember it now. I do remember the visit of the human resources manager—someone I worked closely with—at DHMC. I was conscious enough to understand her updates with a certain degree of humor, but I no doubt did not leave a hopeful impression.

Spaulding Rehabilitation Hospital

I felt aware enough to perceive my transition to Spaulding, a rehab hospital in Boston. Since I remained confined to a bed, I rode from DHMC in an ambulance.

My first taste of a big-city hospital happened on arrival. Though they must have been expecting me, no one knew exactly where I should go. The ambulance crew finally left me in a room on the eighth floor, where head injuries went.

My initial stay at Spaulding didn't last long. I woke up in the middle of the second night some worried faces.

Somehow, my body had destroyed the trach tube, and fragments of it were still inside. And there was, finally, some blood. An ambulance took me to Mass General a few blocks away, where a surgeon removed the shards of plastic from my chest and inserted a new trach tube.

I felt perversely proud that my body had rejected the trach tube. Staff at Spaulding had suctioned me (a very unpleasant procedure that seemed like suffocating) for the first time earlier that day, and I attributed that procedure to my bodily reaction and the trach tube incident, though the suctioning may have been completely unrelated. I spent the next few days at the ICU in Mass General before I eventually moved back to Spaulding.

Not long after I returned to Spaulding, I was packed off to Mass Eye and Ear to have my right eye sewn shut. The procedure was intended to protect the eye (and keep it from drying out) since I couldn't close the eye and the cornea was scratched. The result didn't work very well, and I ended up having the stitches removed a few days later. My wife blocked the vision on my glasses on the right side to help with the distraction. The contact lenses I usually wore extensively were not on the radar.

The routine at Spaulding consisted of someone coming in each morning and writing the day's schedule on a makeshift whiteboard. Each day I had physical therapy (PT), occupational therapy (OT), and therapy for speech and language pathology (SLP). Later, periodic visits from a psychologist began, although these did not appear on my daily schedule. Initially, staff used an electric patient lift (a winch and harness) to get me out of bed and into a wheelchair. Later, I could do the transfer with aid but without the lift.

At Spaulding, I spent all my time either in a wheelchair or in bed. Most of the day (I won't say waking hours since I frequently napped) I spent in a wheelchair. Sitting upright in the chair posed an exertion, and I sometimes slumped over the side.

I often felt nauseated, probably because my balance system had been so damaged. Pressing my head back in the high-back wheelchair seemed to help stabilize things. In bed, things stopped moving so much as long as I laid flat on my back. I threw up once in PT, but generally I managed to hold things down.

I noticed my hearing getting weaker in the first weeks at Spaulding. Perhaps it had been damaged all along, and I just started to notice.

I underwent a full battery of hearing tests at Mass Eye and Ear. The results were not encouraging. I had completely lost hearing on my right side and was not expected to recover any. My left ear had some hearing remaining, but it appeared significantly damaged. I have always loved music, so this news did not thrill me.

Perhaps this is an appropriate point to mention that medical staff never told me a prognosis (at least that I can remember), probably because it was so uncertain. Someone told my wife to expect a full recovery with possibly a bit of a limp when I walked. Somehow I knew that as well; possibly she shared that info with me or I heard someone talking. Whatever the reason, I felt I was underperforming at rehab when functions weren't coming back. That disappointed feeling persisted for months.

Mornings were tough at Spaulding. Before the accident, I

was accustomed to waking early (say, five a.m.) and working out with weights before breakfast. Now, nothing much happened until nine a.m. or so.

I still awoke early. Given the time of year, I awakened in darkness. I would watch for the outside light to start, then observe the sun climbing by watching a shadow on a wall outside the window crawl along. I typically endured seasonal depression due to the lack of light in late fall. Now this depression coupled with the agony of lying in bed unable to do much.

Nighttime did not prove much better. Darkness came early. It hardly mattered, since things quieted early, and most patients were asleep by eight p.m., if not earlier. I felt tired and tended to fall asleep early myself. The problem was that I awoke after a few hours. I remember coughing for what seemed like hours and feeling gripped by terror as I lay there in the darkness unable to move.

Pain was not a serious problem. I had a headache for which I got liquid acetaminophen (Tylenol), which dulled the sensation. In fact, I got everything in liquid form. I had a stomach tube (gastric tube or G-tube) through which I received all my food, water, and medication. The nurse would grind up any pills I needed. Given the trach tube and lack of swallowing function, nothing could be administered by mouth. Like most patients, I got meds twice a day, in the morning and evening.

Nutrition came from small cans (later cartons) that would be fed to the G-tube by a metering pump on a pole. I received liquid food at least twice a day, and the pump would also run slowly overnight. The bed was set at a slant with the head raised to help things go where they were supposed to go.

Despite this feeding schedule, my weight started to fall (probably since I no longer worked out). I went down at least as far as 145 pounds. I saw the look of concern on the faces of staff as they recorded the declining numbers each time.

On the other end, I used a plastic hand urinal to pee and a bedpan to poop. At first, the staff used a condom catheter on me all the time, then later only at night. Once in a while the catheter leaked, necessitating a bed linen change. A few times the G-tube also leaked with the same result. After initial embarrassment, I began to see these things as the staff do: simply necessary (though sometimes messy) biological functions.

Throughout the initial period (several weeks), I wore a cervical collar, which immobilized my neck while my skull knitted back together. Fitting the collar was not easy, and I recall frequent adjustments as well as discomfort. After weeks and multiple X-rays, my skull had knitted, and the collar was finally removed. I felt grateful to be rid of it. In retrospect, I don't know how I endured the weeks in the collar. I have always been somewhat claustrophobic, so the collar must have been difficult to endure.

I still had the trach tube, and removal of that now became my obsession for over a month or so. To help assist my breathing, some sort of humidification system had been used with the trach tube since the beginning (at DHMC). I thought it excessive until the system was removed for a few hours one day. My airways dried out quickly without the added moisture.

I ended up going through half a dozen trach tubes in less than three months. As I explained earlier, the first trach tube got destroyed. Another was removed intentionally by a doctor, then replaced a few hours later because I vomited (which risked my airway).

The weirdest loss of a trach tube occurred when I went to Mass General for a procedure. The doctor removed my trach tube momentarily (intending to put it back in place), then couldn't find it again among the blankets on the table. I did what I could do to help, searching from my back. The doctor never found the missing trach tube and had to install a new one. This substitution only posed a problem since the lost tube was an older model (which worked much better for me) that was probably the last of its kind in the city of Boston (or so I was told). Talk about Murphy's Law!

Finally having the trach tube removed a couple of months into my stay at Spaulding felt like a major victory.

The transition to removal of the trach tube took a few days. The process involved capping the tube for some time and monitoring my oxygen saturation with a pulse oximeter. Initially, I had trouble obtaining enough air for more than a few minutes. Eventually, the capping extended into hours with a target of making it through the whole day.

With the tube capped, I felt terrible—weak, light-headed, heart laboring—at the end of the day. It helped tremendously when I finally recalled feeling this way when my blood sugar fell when I hadn't eaten recently. The awful sensations didn't arise from lack of oxygen but from the need for food!

In a related area, I struggled to communicate. With the initial configuration of the trach tube, the air flowed both ways, preventing any speech, since little air passed my vocal folds. Later, a one-way valve capped the trach tube so that I could exhale through my throat. While this made speech theoretically possible, I remained largely mute.

Besides gestures, I communicated by pointing to letters on a letter board. The process was slow (obviously) but better than nothing.

The problems with this method grew especially acute at night, when nearly all the staff were not native English speakers. I awoke on more than one occasion (for instance, a leaking feeding tube). I remember frantically trying to spell things out and the staff being unable to interpret my wild hand motions at the letter board. It probably didn't help that my right hand had lost much of its coordination. A later test showed that one of my vocal folds remained mostly paralyzed, and speaking intelligibly remains difficult to this day.

I did my PT, OT, and SLP each day. It was discouraging trying to walk or move my left arm or speak, but the staff kept at me and I did not give up.

I was fitted for a custom-made ankle-foot orthotic (or AFO) on my left leg. This brace forced my foot to a horizontal position (I have drop foot) and prevented my left knee from hyperextending. It helped me bear weight on my left leg, though my gait became fairly monstrous (watch an old *Frankenstein* movie).

During this time and the coming months, I became well-acquainted with a suction wand called a Yankauer. Beyond the suctioning of my lungs by catheter that medical personnel did a few times each day (never pleasant), I could use a Yankauer to suction myself in my mouth and throat.

The wand and I became inseparable whenever I lay in bed.

The Yankauer received suction from the house vacuum system at the hospital via a trap. It seemed amazing to me (not necessarily in a good way) that I had so many secretions that ended up in the trap. (Staff didn't seem shocked, so presumably this is normal.) Periodically someone would have to empty the trap, clean the Yankauer, or replace everything. I loved getting a new setup.

I imagine that anyone who has been hospitalized for a significant period of time has stories. My favorite is the weekend that the staff forgot to feed me.

First, it is necessary to understand that weekends in a rehab hospital are far different from weekdays. Regular staff have their own home life, and many are off during the weekends. Thus, a mostly new group (usually with less seniority) is around on weekends. The people at Spaulding did a nice job of trying to get me out of bed on weekends. I often had a session with a cycling trainer in lieu of PT.

Next, remember that I had a G-tube, so feedings were not participatory. Often, I barely knew they were occurring.

That particular Sunday afternoon, I awoke from a nap feeling chilled. (My body historically had trouble staying warm without frequent food.) I also felt a little light-headed as well as tired. My heart seemed to flutter a bit. As I often did, I tried to sort out these signals. On reconstructing the preceding days, I realized that no one had been in to feed me since that Friday.

I buzzed the nurse on duty to explain the problem. She was mortified. Some food was soon delivered (always via the metering pump), so I started to feel better. Suffice it to say, that never happened again.

Throughout my stay, my wife stayed with me most of each day, which helped tremendously. She read to me and ran interference with the staff. With my limited ability to communicate, her help proved vital.

Several times, I bundled up (it was mostly December) in the wheelchair and my wife took me outside to an adjacent park on the Charles River to get some fresh air. A few other times, we took small excursions in the hospital such as down to the cafeteria.

I don't know exactly what went on in my absence at work. (The other employees might have thrown a party to celebrate my sudden departure, though I doubt it.) The one concrete read I had was the quantity of cards and letters that arrived. Some came from quarters where I least expected it (like former employees). Some sent several.

The communications helped me to navigate some dark days. One colleague even asked to visit me. As nice a gesture as it was, I didn't want people to see me in such a sorry state and said no. I still had hopes of returning to a more-or-less normal life.

Nights proved most difficult. I had to sleep on my back. The staff tried to get me off my back to prevent bedsores, but it was painful on my left side. I felt dizzy and nauseated on my right. As I noted previously, I tended to awaken each night. I also got prodded with some regularity during the night. The nurse gave me some sleeping medication each evening, but it wore off after a few hours, and I often awoke in the darkness.

The end result came one night. I don't know what I was thinking (or if I was thinking), but I awoke and tried to get out of bed. My legs were not strong enough to support me, and I crumpled to the floor. I didn't hit my head, but I was not strong enough to move.

I lay there on the cold, hard floor in the darkened room for some period. Time passed slowly. I could hear activity in the corridor, yet I felt incapable (or too embarrassed) to call for help. Staff members eventually found me and lifted me back into bed, checking to make sure I wasn't hurt.

The next day, a new bed appeared (much lower to the ground) and soft mats were placed around it. The objective, of course, was to prevent any injury if I got out of bed again. An alarm was also added that sounded if I tried to get up. I know this was all for my own good, but it forced me to lay in bed with little motion. My sense of being imprisoned increased. My wife stayed over a few nights in the next bed, which helped calm me.

Each of these things separately would have been trying, but here they happened all at once. Perhaps it was inevitable that I would suffer a mental toll.

I stayed stoic for a number of weeks through the vision and hearing issues, cervical collar, and various indignities, yet I could feel my resolve and composure slipping away. One day after several weeks at Spaulding, I told the doctor that I only had a couple more weeks. I meant it in two ways: (1) the time away from work had already seemed long and (2) I knew I wouldn't last much longer in the hospital without some sort of mental breakdown.

The doctor chuckled. I was not trying to be funny. I guess the doctor knew that going back to my old life would never happen.

After a couple more weeks, I began to fray. Though I tried to stay composed, my mind began to break down. I began having even more problems sleeping. I underwent episodes of panic. I began to rave for water (which would have to be administered by G-tube).

The staff at the hospital tried to help me (they must have seen this before), yet the only thing that I knew would matter was medication. I received an SSRI (antidepressant) but the drug would take days or weeks to work. In the meantime, I tried to hold it together.

I had read that soldiers in combat draw off a fixed well of courage. When this well is exhausted, they experience mental issues. I had never really understood this fact in a deep way. Now I felt it firsthand. I don't mean to equate my experience with what veterans and some first responders endure. After all, I was injured entertaining myself, not doing something noble like defending our country or saving lives. Moreover, I lay in a modern hospital surrounded by professionals trying to help me. I merely mean I could now understand the phenomenon of running out of resolve.

Over time, I improved. Perhaps the medication worked. Perhaps I adjusted. Perhaps it was a combination. Whatever happened, I survived. I felt much more mentally frail and had difficult moments, but I continued.

A psychologist regularly visited me at Spaulding, and met separately with my wife. Not surprisingly, some professional assistance with mental health helped.

I think it is common for patients with life-changing injuries to feel despair or to contemplate taking their own life. I certainly went through it. I had dealt with suicidal thoughts many years before, so maybe I was primed for those questions. Perhaps my previous experience also aided me in dismissing the thought of any action. I felt adamant that I would not do anything to hurt myself. I chose to survive not for myself but for my wife and adult son.

The mechanics of suicide would have been challenging in a medical facility focused on preserving my life, but I imagine I could have figured something out. I never chose to do so. I would urge others to choose similarly and dismiss any thoughts of self-harm. If nothing else, tell yourself to wait until circumstances are different. Procrastinating (until such time that a suicidal act again feels like a poor option) may be the best you can do.

Toward the end of my stay (roughly two months) at Spaulding after the trach tube finally came out, the staff began preparing me to transition. I was not ready to go home, but another less-intensive rehab center was available. I began to use a toilet and take a shower instead of receiving a sponge bath. I did not feel pleased to be going to yet another institution, but clearly going home was not a viable option.

Another thing that seemed to accelerate toward the end were blood draws. I had received them occasionally before, but now the frequency increased.

I have never had a fear of needles, and at this point that fact was a good thing. Since the circulation in my left arm is weak, we always used my right arm (despite the fact that it was not numb like the left so I felt the needle). A thing one discovers when having blood drawn frequently: the skill of phlebotomists varies to a surprising degree. Some have no trouble. Others struggle to properly perforate a blood vessel. I think the record for me was getting stuck twelve times by one individual in a single setting before a sample could be drawn.

Near the end, my caregivers tried to involve me in some recreation. I had always been an outdoor sports enthusiast, and Spaulding offered substantial recreation opportunities outside.

But only in better weather. In winter, the cold was not conducive to being outdoors. Instead, the staff brought a three-wheel bike inside and let me ride a little in a hallway. It's hard to describe how great that felt. One might question the sanity of someone getting on a bike after being injured so significantly in a cycling accident. I didn't care.

To add to my overall frustration, my departure from Spaulding was delayed a few days because my white blood cell count had elevated above normal. The doctor told me it could just occur from the excitement of anticipation, but they wanted to hold me to be sure I did not bring an infection to my new location.

Finally, I was cleared, and an ambulance came to take me to Crotched Mountain.

Chapter 4

Crotched Mountain Rehab

For a long time, I struggled to spell *crotched*, often confusing it with *crochet*. This difficulty was odd since I've always been a good speller. I guess the struggle was an indication of just how badly my brain functioned.

As at Spaulding, my introduction to Crotched Mountain was not auspicious. The ambulance crew that transported me had to make a few stops on the campus before unloading me, because my placement seemed uncertain. (I was hardly unexpected. Are all medical facilities difficult to check into?) It was not a great beginning.

After I settled into my room, a nice young member of the staff took my wife and me on a tour. The facility consisted of multiple interconnected buildings making up three sides of a large square. The section where I was housed was in a newish building at the clockwise end of the complex. An enclosed hallway led to a school (my understanding is that Crotched Mountain started as a school for the Deaf) with an athletic area—including a gym and an indoor pool—and a library. Another enclosed hallway connected to a modest hospital at the far counterclockwise position.

This complex was situated out in the country of southern

New Hampshire, many miles from the big city and its hectic pace. The stress of traffic and nonstop activity faded. I realized that I had become a small-town person after many years living in Hanover. I wasn't home, but this felt much closer.

I spent the first few days in a single room. I later realized they put all newcomers in this room to be sure we were not infectious. My wife stayed in a guest house on the campus, since the facility was far removed from an urban area with hotels.

The standard rooms in the head injury unit were spacious doubles, one of which I moved into after a few days. The furniture could be arranged as patients liked, and most people (including me) set up rooms as two separate spaces.

I remained in a hospital bed, with the head raised slightly. The room had the typical hospital panel for each bed, with a call button, vacuum, etc. Initially I used a Yankauer, though eventually that went away. Each bed had windows that had a view of the countryside. I moved rooms occasionally. In my last room, where I stayed the longest, I had a glorious view of Mt. Monadnock. No wonder this felt more homelike than the city.

I remember getting offered a whirlpool bath my first weekend, after only being on-site a day. This may have been intended as a special treat for patients, but I assumed this was routine and had baths every two evenings throughout my stay. (Most patients had morning showers.)

I began to shave myself. Going without shaving was not really an option since I had begun treatment with electrical stimulation on my neck, and the electrodes needed skin contact. The objective was to help me swallow. At Spaulding, someone had always shaved me. Now I began to do it myself.

I have always shaved with a blade, not an electric razor. Not trusting myself to do anything nuanced around my lips with a sharp object, I left a goatee. (I have had a mustache since I was eighteen.) I learned to put on shave cream and manipulate the razor in my right hand and developed the habit of shaving every day to feel less like a patient and more like a functioning member of society. I also tried to brush my teeth each morning even though I was not eating by mouth.

Like the trach tube before, and the cervical collar before that, my obsession turned to ridding myself of the G-tube. Alas, I had no success until long after I went home from Crotched Mountain. The other patients gathered in a communal room for meals. Not me. A staff member administered my liquid nourishment in my room.

I quickly adopted the practice of placing an extra towel on my lap, since the G-tube feedings could be messy on occasion. I still had a slow trickle of liquid food administered by a metering pump at night.

One would think I would start to gain weight with being so sedentary. Nope. I was always one of those people who lost weight when I didn't work out (lost muscle mass, I guess). The trend continued at Crotched Mountain. They weighed me here on a platform while in the wheelchair (they had weighed the chair separately). I didn't know exactly what numbers they measured, but staff didn't seem concerned, so I think my weight had stabilized at a low value.

Shortly after starting me at Crotched Mountain, my wife returned to her job as a teacher. She had always worked four-day weeks and returned to that. On her three-day weekends, she would come down to Crotched Mountain and stay in the guest house. I missed her but got used to being alone.

I no longer had the trach tube, but communicating remained a challenge. For the most part, my speech remained unintelligible. My hearing stayed limited. I continued to use a letter board to spell things out, though I now expanded my use of a computer. I'm sure it won't shock those who have traveled overseas extensively in places without a common language, but one can go a long way by simply smiling and nodding. (The tactic works exceptionally well in a health-care setting where everyone tries to be helpful.)

A nice lounge existed in the unit where patients could socialize, watch TV, and get out of their wheelchairs onto some upholstered furniture. I used the lounge some but not extensively. With my inability to hear or speak, socializing did not work very well. On the TV in my own space, I had captioning set up so that I could understand the programs.

As at Spaulding, I had frequent sessions of PT, OT, and SLP. Most of the sessions occurred in conventional therapy gyms or the patient's room. One time I had a physical therapy session in the swimming pool. The pool had a variable depth floor and a ramp so that a pool wheelchair could descend right into the water. Unfortunately, my balance was so messed up that I tended to fall over if I didn't hang on to the side of the pool. That ranks as the first and only therapy I have had in the water.

Crotched Mountain had a psychologist as well. I met with her regularly, but I didn't have a crisis as before at Spaulding. I don't know what drugs they administered. I probably still took the antidepressant.

I went through a progression of walkers, beginning with a rollator that I could lean on (placing a bunch of weight on it) and ending with a lightweight aluminum walker where I stood more upright. They also had a standing frame that I came to use twice daily so I could get accustomed to putting weight on my legs. Therapists had me do sit-to-stand exercises. Despite all this, my go-to where I spent most of my time remained a wheelchair.

Being back in rural New Hampshire in winter, of course, meant snowstorms. On especially bad days (there were only a few), the place would partially shut down with no or limited PT, OT, and SLP. These snow days never bothered me, as I had long been accustomed to them as part of life in the north.

On one occasion, I traveled to Mass Eye and Ear in Boston for another evaluation of my right eye, which was mostly blind. The conclusion was not favorable; I would have to get used to having vision only on my left.

For this trip, I rode in a wheelchair in a van instead of on my back in an ambulance. I felt less seriously injured by being able to sit up.

I recall the long drive. I was then coughing up lots of phlegm, thus consuming plenty of tissues. I remember the van encountered a serious traffic accident in the dark on a small two-lane road on the way back that delayed us considerably. Despite trying to conserve them, I ran short of tissues because of the delay.

Over time, I learned to use the bathroom on my own. I still had a condom catheter at night, but during the day I managed by myself using either a plastic hand urinal and/ or grab bars. I learned to have a schedule for using the bathroom, not just go "on feel" as I had before my skull fracture. Aides still monitored me, though I needed less and less help.

I had extensive SLP therapy primarily aimed at getting me to safely swallow. To me, swallowing had never been something I had to think about. It simply happened. Now, it required intense focus to prevent aspirating into my lungs.

I had begun electrical stimulation of my throat muscles at Spaulding, and it continued at Crotched Mountain. My understanding was that the typical course of treatment by electrical stimulation was about two months. I think I eventually endured—no, the treatment was not pleasant, but I desperately wanted to get better—sessions for over a year extending into my outpatient care.

At first, the SLP therapist only had me try bottled water. I learned to make the rear part of my tongue shift back and down to aid swallowing. After a couple months of work, I had my first barium swallow study at a nearby hospital. In this, you attempt to consume various things that have barium as a tracer. They monitor you by fluoroscopy (continuous X-ray). Since barium is a heavy metal (a nontoxic one), it shows up clearly in the images.

Though hopeful going in, I failed the barium swallow study. I was not swallowing effectively, risking aspiration and my airway. Back to work we went. I know the SLP therapist at one point told my wife that I would probably need the G-tube permanently. I might get to the point where I could take a little food for mouth feel, but I would still need the G-tube for nutrition, a depressing prospect.

One big success came after I had been at Crotched Mountain a couple months. I had been plagued by muscle-tension headaches throughout my adult life. After the accident, I had endured constant pain in my head. I assumed pain was part of having a head injury.

I don't remember precisely why, but one day one of the nurses decided to try to help. Maybe I had complained of a constant headache once too often. This particular nurse—I can still picture her—knew pressure-point massage, so she offered to search for a spot. She rapidly narrowed her search to a place on my right shoulder blade. She could feel the muscle there knotted up.

I was skeptical that anything so removed from my head could matter, but the nurse insisted on coming back to do what she could. Despite my misgivings, I was in too much constant pain to argue. What could it hurt anyway? She applied intense finger pressure to the knot several times over a couple days. The pressure felt painful, but we kept at it.

After a few treatments over a couple of days, the knot relaxed, and my headache vanished. Apparently, the muscle involved runs up the neck and around the skull. I am guessing that the healing of my broken collarbone resulted in the knot. Amazingly, the headaches never returned. That outcome has led me to experiment with all manner of alternative treatments since.

To try to improve my limited hearing, my wife and I saw an outpatient audiologist at Crotched Mountain. She fitted me with a hearing aid on the left. (On the right, I remained completely deaf.) The aid allowed me to hear things I couldn't before—including people approaching from behind, so I didn't startle as readily—but as any person with a hearing instrument will tell you, it also amplified noises.

I can't hear on the right, but that doesn't mean there is

silence there. I hear my pulse on the right, rather loudly. Coupled with the noises on my left, the end result was a cacophony of sound and no peace. After a few days, I returned the hearing aid.

At one point, staff replaced my G-tube. For the uninitiated, a G-tube penetrates your abdomen to get into your stomach. It has at least two fittings. When the tube is implanted, one fitting is used to inflate a balloon to hold the tube in your stomach. It is not touched until removal. The other fitting(s) takes in the liquid food, water, and ground medication.

I had expected a cautious process of deflating the balloon, then carefully extracting the tube. Instead, it was a fairly violent process. The balloon was mostly deflated, and the extraction involved a swift and forceful jerk. A new tube was immediately poked into the aperture since my body's healing would start to close off the path right away.

In addition to the near-constant attention from my wife, I had a few other visitors. Her older brother and his wife came regularly.

Two friends from back in high school, Kurt and Nick, came to see me. We had done a reunion bicycle trip shortly before my accident. The three of us had taken bike trips together in high school and college. We had previously done a reunion trip—having a great time—a few years before. My injury meant that we would never again carve out time from our jobs and families to cycle together.

A colleague from work and her husband also stopped to see me. I gave them a tour of the facility. Though I imagine I spoke mostly unintelligibly, they were nice and acted like they understood what I said.

In addition to the visitors—not many, since Crotched Mountain was remote to where I lived in Hanover—I did get plenty of mail. By this time, I could read moderately well. I also became more active on the computer.

A big part of my time at Crotched Mountain focused on exercise and recreation. Not long after I arrived, my wife helped me get on a glider, sort of like a cross-country ski machine, which I loved but only used a few times. One of the staff organized a yoga class. The group did sitting motions from our wheelchairs mostly. We must have been a sight, though anything to enhance flexibility was no doubt helpful.

A key advance involved staff putting me on a recumbent stepper. I started off for just a few minutes, eventually going for twenty-plus minutes. I would push myself so that I actually got warm. I wouldn't quite break a sweat, yet the exertion felt good. The ability to exercise made me feel like recovery was in progress.

While the snow stayed in good shape, my wife and a group of volunteers took me downhill skiing a couple times. I had never, of course, been in a sit-ski, but the instructors made it easy. They even took me over a small jump, though I asked them not to do it again since the landing felt too jarring for my head (sit-skis have some but not enough suspension). Speeding down the mountain in the fresh air felt great but left me wishing for the old days of skiing on my own.

As early spring came on, the staff started putting me on a three-wheeled bike to ride indoors through the facility. (My wife must have told them how much I loved cycling.) The facility was fully connected indoors, so I could ride all the way around the three sides of the square without going outside, maybe a half mile each way. In one location, the bike even fit in an elevator to ride down to the ground floor. I'm sure I rode very slowly—a staff member could walk briskly beside me—but I felt great being in the saddle again.

As the weather warmed and the snow receded, my wife could take me outside in my wheelchair for a trip around the campus. One day they took me outside on the bike. Patients frequently went outside on a deck at midday to enjoy the sun. Things felt springlike, with the sense of rebirth that happens each year.

All this time my therapies continued. The PT focused on my walking and balance (which improved but never got very good). The OT worked on a variety of things. In addition to the usual OT objectives like making my hands function better, the therapists tried to help with my balance. I remained hopeful that things would improve. SLP kept up with the e-stim to get me eating and drinking, but to no avail.

Near the end of my stay at Crotched Mountain, I spent a couple weekends at home to help ease the coming transition. The drive back to Hanover as a passenger felt surreal. I had seen the route on a map and heard my wife describe it but had never seen it in person. The impression of unreality grew at home. I knew everything, yet it felt like I was seeing it for the first time.

These trips required lots of preparation for my wife. She had to get a shower bench, a plastic handheld urinal, and a foam wedge pillow for me. She had to help give me my liquid food and grind up my pills for the G-tube. Thanks to all of her preparation, no significant snags occurred.

Once back at Crotched Mountain in those final weeks, I

researched recumbent trikes on my laptop for riding outside when I got home.

Finally the day came to go home for good. Although looking forward to being home, unlike leaving DHMC and Spaulding, I felt less impatient to depart the institution's routines. After the inauspicious beginning, I had grown genuinely fond of Crotched Mountain[1] and could see myself there for a while, doing my therapies, watching my captioned TV, and getting my liquid nourishment. In addition—despite the transition weekends that had gone well—the prospect of being without trained medical staff only a buzz away scared me a little.

Maybe those feelings are a tribute to the people and facilities at Crotched Mountain. Maybe I had changed. Whatever the reason, the time had come to move forward.

---

1 The brain injury unit at Crotched Mountain closed a few years ago.

Chapter 5

Home Again ... And Outpatient

"There's no place like home."

Dorothy said that in the *Wizard of Oz*, so the concept of home seems magical for nearly everyone. It was for me. After being away in institutions for months save the two recent weekend visits, home felt familiar yet foreign to me when I finally arrived there.

Same town. Same house (with a new master bath). The drawers and their contents in the bedroom were even the same. Yet the sense of being in someone else's life felt almost palpable. The impression of strangeness probably reflected my vantage point from a wheelchair as well.

Many things at home remained just as I had left them in the fall. I recognized them, but they felt like they belonged to another person. This sense of feeling like a different person persisted in many contexts, though largely subsided after a few weeks. We had partly moved to our lakeside cottage shortly before my accident. The fact that my possessions were scattered between the in-town house and the cottage probably exacerbated my confusion.

The time was May. The late fall, winter, and early spring had passed while I was away. Summer stood poised to launch.

My wife had prepared extensively for my homecoming the previous weekends. Those preparations became my norm now that I was home to stay. She had invested in a foam wedge so that I didn't have to sleep flat. She had picked up a plastic hand urinal to use at night. Farewell to nighttime catheters. I had wooden ramps to enter and exit the house in my chair.

The master bath remodeling that had been underway at the time of my accident had long been completed. A couple of grab bars and a shower bench were in place for me to function.

Perhaps I should describe the house. It is a ranch with an exposed basement or lower level. The rooms I use most—kitchen, family room, master suite, and a garage—are upstairs on the main level. On the lower level are my gym and home office, along with other bedrooms and another garage (under the main one upstairs; we mostly use it to store things).

A narrow, steep stairway with a sharp turn near the bottom connects the two levels. In good weather, I can move between floors outside. I exit the upper garage (where a ramp is) in a wheelchair, roll down a paved driveway, and reenter the house on the lower level via the lower garage (and another ramp). If the weather doesn't allow that, I can navigate the stairs on my feet or butt, using railings on each side and someone holding a gait belt.

I had barely been home when an ambulance had to haul me to the emergency room because I couldn't urinate. The problem was only temporary, and I got back to a regular bathroom schedule quickly.

The ambulance came one more time early that summer.

The lip at the edge of our garage upstairs was precipitous, and I casually rode the wheelchair off it without thinking. I crashed and smashed my glasses into my eyebrow above my left eye socket.

The wound bled voluminously. I remember laying on the asphalt of the driveway watching a red river stream down. Though I had read of "streets running with blood" historically before, I thought it was just a literary reference. In this incident, I learned better. Head wounds bleed a lot.

By the time the rescue squad arrived (just a few minutes), I'd remounted the chair, and most of the bleeding had stopped. The ambulance crew helped clean me up and applied a small bandage, and I decided not to go to the hospital.

My wife hired an aide (a licensed nursing assistant, or LNA) to stay with me during the day and when she traveled. This person would help me walk with my rollator, do my exercises, arrange my meals, and drive me to appointments. The LNA kept an eye on me. I initially felt not quite sure how to react to this person in my house. Was it a guest? Over time (and several aides) I learned a home aide functioned as just a helper, but it took a while.

I still had the G-tube and could not take food or drink by mouth. One of my colleagues from work had ginned up a contraption to hold the apparatus so that I could feed myself. I migrated to three liquid meals per day of two cartons each with no feeding at night. I also supplemented the liquid diet with water (administered by G-tube), especially in hot weather.

I resumed PT, OT, and SLP as an outpatient shortly after arriving home. I took PT and OT from a private company (where I still do PT today) and SLP at DHMC. I'll describe my progression at PT later. OT officially ended after a few months when I stopped progressing, though I still do some continuing work with my hands as part of PT even today.

The SLP therapy focused on getting me eating and drinking by mouth. I had at least weekly appointments where again we tried electrical stimulation. Despite using the e-stim at full power (really not fun) and practicing exercises at home, I still failed a barium swallow study. I remained on the G-tube. Depressing.

In addition to the therapies, I also went to massage regularly. I didn't experience a dramatic change again like I had at Crotched Mountain with my head pain, but the treatment helped me to loosen up. I felt like a limp noodle afterward.

Shortly after arriving home, I ordered a recumbent trike. I felt excited to cycle again, and my wife hauled me to a number of local trails where traffic would not be an issue.

I bought a normal recumbent trike (nothing specially adaptive), a delta with one wheel in front, which made it easy for me to climb on. Unfortunately, the trike also proved easy to fall off or to capsize. I tipped going around corners. I fell off a sidewalk. I hit a small rock. I ran off into the woods on a rail trail trying to avoid a young child. Though the crashes were at low speed and I wasn't hurt, hitting the ground is not a recommended tactic for recovering from head injuries. My wife, riding behind to watch over me, was horrified.

As for the cause of the mishaps, I don't know whether it was the fact that on a delta the two wheels were behind me (out of my vision) or that I had such weak balance that

I couldn't sense bad situations or that the trike's center of gravity was too high or some combination of these factors. Clearly, something needed to change.

My weight stayed low. Photos of me at that time show how skinny I had become. I had never been overweight, but now I looked almost emaciated. At least I felt fine.

I got a text-to-speech app on a tablet computer to help me communicate. Using the app seemed cumbersome, but I could save phrases and short talks that I would use frequently. Given that my speech remained unintelligible most of the time, the app seemed a necessity. When people from work visited, they nodded as if they understood me when I spoke, though I'm sure they did not. It took major effort and lots of concentration to speak, even badly.

I returned to work for a visit that summer. Everyone was incredibly nice, but clearly I was not ready to start working again. Seeing my old office (also untouched since my sudden departure) felt surreal. Same desk. Same photos. Same chair. I recognized it as mine, yet felt like an intruder.

By the end of that first summer home, things had lapsed into a recurring pattern. I got up and tried to work out in my home gym downstairs. As mentioned before, for decades previous to my accident, I had worked out in the early morning, and I tried to recapture that sense of normalcy. I did my speech exercises and went to PT. I took a nap. (I always felt tired.) I had my liquid meals. We stopped the SLP since it seemed to do no good. (I didn't miss the electrical stimulation.) As at Crotched Mountain, I watched lots of television. (I even found the same oldies channel.)

In late August, changes were afoot. Forward again. My wife headed back to school. The aide who had been with me all summer departed. I started riding a different trike, a tadpole (two wheels in front and much lower to the ground) that we rented from a disabled sports organization.

In September, I started with a new outpatient SLP therapist at a small community hospital (Alice Peck Day, or APD) in the next town. (My wife remained persistent in hoping I would improve.) The therapist at APD had also suffered a TBI almost twenty years before. She quickly observed that I tended to cough, which she took as a positive sign that I could try to clear my airway. (Previously, I had been conditioned to think that coughing was a negative. The coughing still meant that food and drink were trying to enter my lungs, but the new revelation to me was that coughing meant my body was clearing them.) In short order, this new therapist had me taking a little food and drink by mouth.

I also got a new aide, one who would stay with me until late spring. I grew close to this woman, who structured my time effectively. Many of the routines I still follow were established with her. I remember that one of the first things this aide asked me was whether I had a "do not resuscitate" order. I knew why she asked, but the question still felt a little disconcerting coming from the person who was supposed to take care of me. (Fortunately, except for that time in the ambulance right after the initial crash, I have not needed any resuscitation.)

I had gotten my own tadpole trike and then, in October, my brother and his wife and my friend Kurt and his wife came to accompany me and my wife on a thirty-mile charity ride. I was extremely slow, but I finished, a major victory. Staying hydrated meant taking water through my G-tube at rest breaks (weird but workable), though I was able to swallow a few sips of beer at the finish.

Throughout that winter, I continued to work with the SLP therapist at APD. I slowly upped the food and water I could take by mouth. We also worked on my speech. She made a key insight that my soft palate had trouble closing completely, leading to a very nasal tone especially when I tried to speak loudly, which I often did in order to hear myself. Knowing this, I tried to reduce volume so that air pressure did not overwhelm my weak palate muscles.

I also began acupuncture treatment to determine if that would help. The doctor of traditional Chinese medicine was very nice, but the sessions ultimately did not make a noticeable difference.

That November and again that winter in February, my wife and I traveled out to Wisconsin to visit my mother, who had just moved into an assisted living facility. The November trip went fine, but in February we hit a bad snowstorm.

I managed to dislodge my G-tube at the airport on the way out in February, which wasn't a total disaster since our flight had been canceled anyway. I had the G-tube replaced at DHMC, and we made the trip to Wisconsin a few days later.

Traveling with a G-tube provided a number of challenges. I remember my wife had to pack almost an entire suitcase with my liquid food for just a few days away.

By spring that year (eighteen months after my accident), I could eat more and more by mouth, but my walking hadn't improved markedly. I still spent most of the time in a wheelchair and used a rollator on those limited occasions when I tried to walk, always with an attendant.

One episode that spring pointed out why I liked the

SLP therapist so much. I had yet another barium swallow study scheduled. I felt more confident since I was eating and drinking regularly by mouth at my therapy sessions.

At the outset of the test, I did poorly, to the extent that the physician conducting the test wanted to halt because of worry about my aspiration. My SLP therapist insisted we continue. She had seen me consume food for months with no ill effects. As I took more of the barium-laced food, a curious thing happened. My swallowing improved. Later, my therapist said she had never seen someone's swallowing stabilize in a positive way over the course of a test. Perhaps, she speculated, my throat muscles needed a warm-up.

As she recommended, I still warm up a little by drinking a few sips of water before a meal. I am so thankful that she pushed us on during that study. Otherwise, I might still be using a G-tube today.

I visited my brother's family in Tucson (they have since moved to Wisconsin where we grew up). The warm weather felt very nice. We rented a tadpole trike similar to what I had in Hanover so I could ride (slowly; everyone was so patient).

One big thing in spring occurred when, unprompted, two therapists independently told me that I didn't need the ankle-foot orthotic anymore. I happily abandoned that device. To this day, my left knee hyperextends and my left foot still tends to drop, though I fight those issues.

Another change over those months occurred when I shed most of the medications. I took a number of medications each day when I first arrived home. One thing I learned, which may or may not be true: doctors seem happy to prescribe new things but loathe to cancel medications that other doctors order. The net result, of course, is that the list of medications gets longer over time as new things are added, but nothing is ever dropped.

I don't have a problem taking medications I need, but I prefer to go without. Almost everything has a side effect of some sort, though it may be minor or worth the trouble. To eliminate medications, I began to phase them out gradually. Some were easy, others more difficult.

The most difficult drug to eliminate was a medication I had "prescribed" for myself: meclizine. Though I had originally requested it just so I would avoid motion sickness on the transfer from Spaulding to Crotched Mountain in the ambulance, the medication had become part of the suite of drugs I took every day. (I had had positive experiences with over-the-counter meclizine for preventing seasickness before my accident.) Phasing the meclizine out without inducing too much dizziness took time. Like taking it in the first place, the responsibility for ending the medication belonged solely to me.

In addition to all the other changes in that first year of being home, we tried to address my hearing and vision issues. I met with an audiologist at DHMC who equipped me with two ear-mounted devices. For my right ear, which hears nothing externally, she gave me an aid that sends sound by radio to my left side. On my left side, I have more of a conventional hearing aid that amplifies external sound. The device also receives the audio from the right and puts it into my left ear. Both appear visually like a typical behind-the-ear aid. After less than a week, I managed to lose one of the devices. We replaced it, but I use the devices only infrequently due to the constant noise on my right side from my pulse.

On vision, things were more complicated. I ended up going in for outpatient surgery at a hospital in Concord, NH, to place a small weight in my right eyelid and partially sew the eye shut. This procedure permits the right eye to close.

The vision on the right is mostly gone, because the cornea has been fouled by blood vessel ingrowth (imagine trying to look through waxed paper). Several opthamologists evaluated me for a cornea transplant. The conclusions were uniformly negative about the prospects in my case. On the left, I experience nystagmus, or spatial jitter—that is, my left eye jerks around slightly and constantly—making it hard to focus.

When my G-tube popped out again in early June, I already ate and drank well enough to forego having it replaced. I rejoiced. Finally, I was free of the G-tube.

I haven't suffered from malnutrition or dehydration. Between working out and solid food, I'm back at about 180 pounds and, like many other people, have to watch things to avoid gaining too much weight. I still cough and eat slowly, but at least I'm eating. In warm weather, I need to drink plenty of extra water.

The subsequent years have not been as eventful. The second part of this account discusses them by topic.

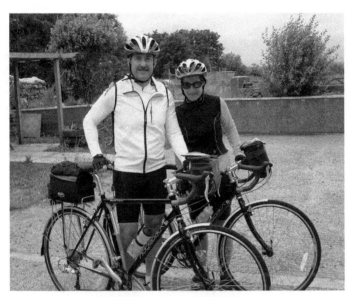

My wife and I in Northern Ireland three months before the accident.

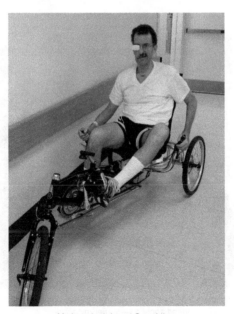

My happiest day at Spaulding.

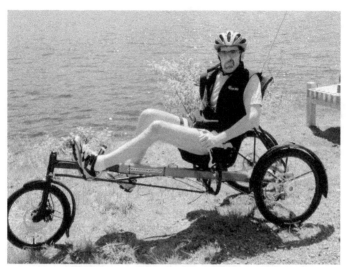

Home again after months in hospitals and rehab centers. Note how skinny I am. This was my first trike, a delta, shortly before one of several capsizes which upset my wife and risked my recovery.

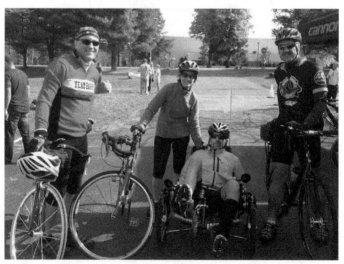

Completing a 30-mile event with my wife, brother, and long-time friend about a year after my accident.

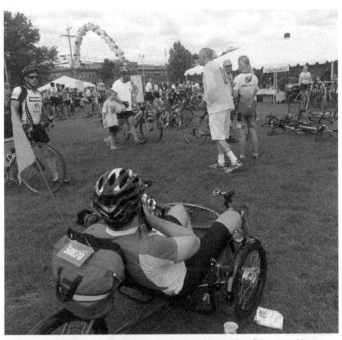

Exhausted after my first 50-mile event about 20 months after my accident.

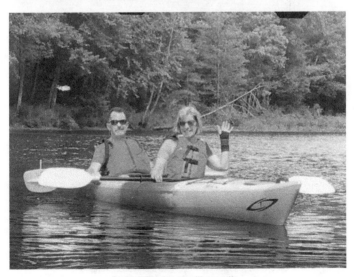

In a tandem kayak with my wife.

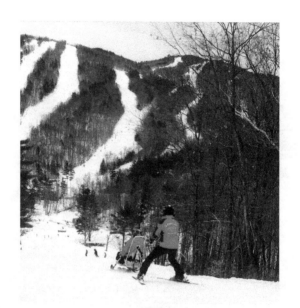

Skiing with an instructor. Note the outriggers on my hands, which I couldn't use effectively.

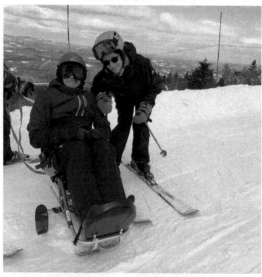

On the slopes with my wife. Note the fixed outriggers on the sled, which work much better for me.

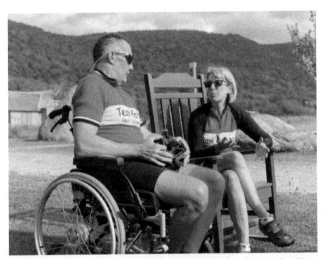

My wife and I were interviewed after Day 1 on a three-day bicycle trip with a disabled group in the White Mountains.

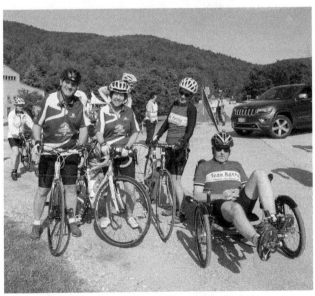

At the start of a 40-mile event with my wife and volunteers.

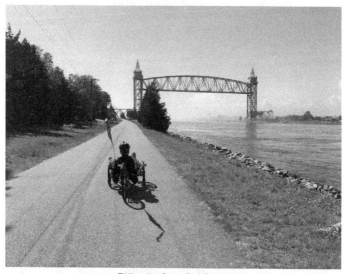
Riding the Cape Cod Canal.

Part 2

Slipping Into a New Normal

Chapter 6

The Pseudo Steady-State

"Acceptance, yes; surrender, no."

That sage piece of advice came from my SLP therapist at APD, who also had a brain injury many years prior. I've never forgotten those words.

From a casual perspective, my life seems pretty static. I remain in a wheelchair. I still have weakness and numbness on the left side, notably my arm and leg. I'm still blind on the right and visually impaired on the left. My hearing also remains similar (deaf on the right and impaired on the left). My face continues to sag on the right.

Yet the casual perspective misses the daily struggle and small victories. So any impression of stasis is wrong.

I have many of the same issues as people everywhere. I have to eat and sleep, though not too much of either. I need exercise. I have work (of a sort) to do. I seek to be entertained. At the same time, I need to battle some things that are unique to my disabled situation.

I continue to go to PT once or twice a week. The therapists there help me try to walk with a rollator. I'm not super-steady though I rarely need help to keep from falling.

After years of work, I sometimes walk with a cane with

a therapist holding on tightly, since a fall here is very likely without help. I also have a series of upper body exercises that I go through in their gym and some OT exercises for my left hand. At the conclusion of each appointment, I do a long aerobic session (forty minutes) on a recumbent stepper machine.

The effort at PT is not completely in vain. My walking has improved, and I can now travel much further than I used to do. Similarly, my pace on the stepper has increased markedly over the years. (Being an engineer who needs to quantify everything, I track my progress in a spreadsheet.) The changes might be small to the uninitiated, but they are very real to me and my therapists. I have gotten occasional comments from strangers, so I know the changes are not completely unnoticed by others.

At home, I have a gym in the lower level of the house. I work out with weights once or twice a week. I can tell that staying strong helps with getting around in a wheelchair. I have a set of parallel bars for practicing walking in my home gym. I try to use them a few times a week. The bars are connected to (and terminate at) a wall so that I can position my wheelchair at the open end of the bars and work by myself. In winter, my trike gets mounted to a trainer in the gym so that I can continue cycling.

I have no expectations that I will eventually walk on my own again. My limited understanding is that one's balance depends on three interacting systems: the inner ear (at least on my right messed up badly), vision (again not working on my right and weak on my left; I imagine the nystagmus is also troublesome), and proprioception (the position of your body in space by sensing joint position; also not functioning well for me, especially on the left). Of the three, I know I rely on proprioception a bunch since I have markedly increased difficulty balancing whenever one foot is out of contact with the floor. My guess is that I slowly conditioned my brain to use this one flawed modality.

In addition to problems with the main balance sensors, I may also have damage to the balance center in my brain. I do some standing exercises each day and have trained myself to stand without holding on for short periods of time if I focus, but I know that this process has limits. Yet it still gives me a daily read on what to expect throughout the day.

I have a similar experience with talking. I do some reading out loud each day (as my SLP therapist at APD advised long ago), and my speech has moved beyond the unintelligible-all-the-time phase to the point where most people can understand me if I concentrate. (They have to concentrate, too, I imagine.) I often remain too loud. I still frequently have to rely on my wife or son to translate, but not as frequently. I'll keep working on my speech even though I know it will never be great.

Voice command seems to be a popular feature of technology today (like Siri and Alexa). Though these tools might seem ideal for a disabled person, I don't imagine I will ever be using a voice-activated device when my speech is already so hard for healthy humans to understand. The rapid advances in computers may make that possible someday.

The lesson in all of this is to keep working, whether it's on physical or not-so-physical things. The gains may be small, but they do add up over time to make it worthwhile. I recognize that this continuing focus is not easy. I certainly encounter times when I want to skip something, but the dogged pursuit of what may seem like ephemeral goals does often pay off eventually.

Perhaps it's useful to summarize my various disabilities here before going on to various other topics. I've already described my vision (blind on the right; nystagmus on the left) and hearing (deaf on the right; tinnitus and significant loss on the left).

In fact, it's easy to track most things using my neck as the divider: below the neck most impairment is on the left; above the neck, issues are mostly on the right. There are a few exceptions like my outer ears (pinnae): numb on left, feeling on right. This instance seems particularly strange since it is opposite to my hearing loss and the other numbness is on the right side of my face. I suppose someone who knows anatomy well would know exactly why there is this pattern (that is, which specific nerves were disrupted), but it doesn't really matter in practice.

I remain numb and weak on the left side. The extremely sharp dividing line between left and right sides has faded a bit since I was first injured (the line used to be only a couple millimeters), but the overall difference continues. I have lost some coordination on the right, but it seems normal in comparison to the left.

Probably the best comparison I can make on the left is that it feels similar to when your arm falls asleep when contorted in some unnatural position for a while. That feeling of numbness pertains to my entire left side all of the time. I can flex my hand and move my leg some, yet there's little strength. I can feel vibration on my left but not temperature.

I should also mention that the little finger on my

left hand is permanently partially curled. I believe it was injured in the original accident, then healed in its current configuration while the rest of my left arm was mostly static. I work frequently on trying to restore the finger to a normal position. The finger is better, though still far from normal.

I am fortunate that I am in no excruciating pain. My left side aches constantly, but no sharp pain is present.

The old adage that nerves and pain remind you not to hurt yourself is true. I need to pay attention to my left side to ensure it does not get injured since pain is not present, at least not immediately. One might think that this makes things like needle sticks for blood draws simple and painless. Unfortunately, my circulation on the left remains weak, so I get most procedures done on the right side, where I still have full feeling. If I get a cut on the left side, the only way I know it is there is by spotting blood.

My autonomic nervous system is somewhat messed up. Although I continue to breathe and my heart keeps beating, some other things don't work right. A good example is temperature control on my left side. I can't consciously sense temperature on that side, but it may go deeper than that. Frequently my left leg feels cold to the touch (as sensed by my functioning right side), yet at other times my left leg gets almost too warm, way different than my right leg. Thus, the thermoregulation of the left leg clearly has been disrupted.

I have few scars associated with the accident, other than the significant divot in the side of my head. (My hair grows asymmetrically now.) At the base of my throat is a depression where the trach tube went. As far as facial appearance, my right eye appears clouded and misaligned, and my face droops on the right.

The most unusual thing about me—though you'd need my shirt off to tell—is that it looks as if I have two belly buttons. One navel we all have from being in the womb. The second comes from the spot where the G-tube was placed to access my stomach. (In a sense, both ports existed for similar reasons.)

All told, much is not working properly. The glass half-full perspective is that much of my body continues to function, at least mostly. The response to either view is the same: keep driving forward.

Chapter 7

Everyday Life

"**I**s there such a thing as a normal day?"

I've often asked myself this question.

Before the accident, my life was full of daily changes and objectives. That hasn't changed since becoming disabled. Despite the constant variation, there are common threads that run through my days.

A Day in the Life . . . Sort Of

In understanding my life now, I think it is helpful to examine a typical day, at least the common elements.

I wake early and usually rise a bit before six a.m. Given total freedom, I tend to awake when it starts to get light, leading to earlier mornings in the summer and later mornings in the dark of winter.

Of course, I typically don't enjoy complete freedom. The cats (we have two) tend to get up to play around five a.m. My wife must rise early (5:45-ish) to get to work during the school year. Thus, I am usually up by six a.m. even in the darkest stretches. I don't feel great getting up these days (does anyone?), though not as bad as I used to feel in the morning in the first months after the accident. I guess the medications I took in those days did have an impact, and losing them has been beneficial in at least this one respect.

I am able to transfer from my bed to the wheelchair without help, and my wife usually gets me some breakfast. I am able to eat and drink fairly normally now, though it helps to focus and go slow. I still sometimes cough, but I haven't been treated for aspiration pneumonia, so I must be doing OK.

I try to read part of the day's paper during breakfast. Reading while eating was once impossible (and still can be slow), but I can do it now. Sometimes, I do have to set aside the reading and focus on the eating, yet mostly it works.

I no longer have aides.

After my wife leaves for work (about 6:50 a.m.), I use the master bath to shower and shave. I am fortunate in that I can maneuver in the bathroom on my own with the help of grab bars and the counter. I use a shower chair to support me in the shower and can stand at the sink (with a good handhold or something to lean on) for ten minutes or so. I brush my teeth with an electric toothbrush.

I still shave with a blade each day to keep up that normalcy. I have an electric beard trimmer that I use twice a week.

Speaking of grooming, my wife cuts my hair at least monthly. When I was in rehab, the ladies at the barber shop sent me a card, an unexpected moment because I assumed I was anonymous. I guess they quizzed my son, who I often went with. Since home, they were most accommodating when an aide took me in, but getting clipped at home is very convenient. My wife also has to clip my toenails. I can do my own fingernails.

I can dress myself and tie my own shoes, though it is slow. I wear elastic-waist shorts and a T-shirt all year since they are easy to deal with and don't make me feel hemmed in. In the cool months, I add a sweatshirt to stay (moderately) warm. During really frigid weather (this is northern New England), I sometimes break down and wear sweatpants, but not often.

After my morning rituals in the master bath and bedroom, I begin the day with standing exercises at a counter in the kitchen. These exercises consume ten to fifteen minutes and give me an early read on whether it will be a good, fair, or poor day for balance. Like most folks, I have good and bad days, and it helps to know which is on tap.

I have tried to divine what makes a day bad or good; find the pattern. My physical therapists have tried as well, asking me questions about how I'm feeling and any recent exercise, trying to connect my varying balance with something. None of us has had luck so far. We know the obvious things like getting too tired, which is clearly an issue, though that seems only part of it.

My favorite theory about good and bad days is that I am responding to small perturbations in my health, for instance, subclinical viral infections like colds. I know that full-blown illnesses hit very hard now. Perhaps my immune system needs to rev up to address smaller threats on a more frequent basis and that takes away from my ability to do other things. At least it's a theory.

Remember my walking balance going awry with an aide? I had just gotten a flu shot. In fact, my balance turns rocky each year when I get a flu shot. These cases are consistent with my theory of some connection to my immune system.

After standing, I next move to the family room and my usual spot on the sofa. I can transfer fairly readily. In cool weather I use a blanket to cover my legs (recall, I wear shorts) when on the sofa.

On the sofa, I retrieve my laptop computer. My first step on the computer is to create my daily to-do list. This list not only contains the things I need to do every day (like standing), it also lists the activities I intend to accomplish that particular day. Like many people, I kept a daily to-do list at the office before my accident. I had one at home on the weekends as well. I continue that practice now. I may be disabled, but I still have many things to do.

Among the things I enter on the list almost every day is some form of exercise and something to do with the kitchen. I don't work out each day (PT or in my gym) since it would lead to exhaustion. I learned the hard way years ago that rest is important, too. Even before my injuries, I had to force myself to take periodic layoffs or face creeping exhaustion. I have always liked working in the kitchen and continue that now.

In addition to my standing exercises, I do a few other things every day: reading out loud, stretching, and meditating. As noted earlier, my SLP therapist at APD recommended reading out loud as a way to improve my speech, and the tactic has worked to some degree. Initially, I used a sound amplifier to help hear nuances in my pronunciation. Now, I usually don't bother. Reading out loud is slow but forces me to concentrate on the sounds I am making.

Stretching is something we should all do, and I did some stretches before my accident as part of my workout routine. Now, stretching has become critical to preserving my quality of life. Much of my stretching focuses on the left side. Without regular attention, my muscles on the left contract and start to limit my range of motion. This process has become an everyday ritual. If I skip a day, I can feel the spasticity growing on my left side, making it more difficult to move.

I took up meditation fairly recently. I initially intended to address anxiety in conjunction with medications. Though it helps with that, meditation helps me focus on many things. I was already far more mindful than in my pre-accident days (I must concentrate to do many things), but meditating promotes this state of mind.

In good weather, I normally sit outside in late morning for about ten minutes to get some sun. (In winter, I will sit in front of a window on sunny days.) Since I don't apply sunscreen, I carefully monitor the time. In addition to the sun exposure, I relish the chance to be in the fresh air.

Much of my day is devoted to "working." This takes the form of physically going into the office (before I retired), writing, preparing things in the kitchen, or conducting research online.

As mentioned earlier, I tire easily and need a nap each day. Perhaps the fatigue results from fighting my muscle contractions all the time. Perhaps I don't sleep as soundly at night as I think I do. Perhaps I am lazy. I typically nap for roughly thirty minutes sitting up on the sofa after lunch, sometimes in the company of a cat.

I get myself lunch. (Typically my wife leaves a sandwich for me.) I either work out in my home gym or go to PT a couple times a week in the afternoon. If not, that's more time to work.

You'll note that I don't mention television. After watching it frequently when I first got home, I try to limit my tube time now. I'd rather read, work, or do a puzzle. It's not as if I never watch TV, just not all the time. I have a big-screen TV in my home gym, so I do watch quite a bit while working out.

Bedtime for me falls at roughly 9:30 p.m. I am able to get myself ready for bed on my own. Once in bed, I sleep on my right side, since that represents the only real option. Back-sleeping results in some form of apnea. Laying on my left side for more than a few minutes is too painful. The disadvantage of sleeping on my right is that it pins down the good side of my body and can make me feel anxious. In the first year or two at home, I sometimes struck out in my dreams, which was hard on my wife, but I haven't done that for a while.

Functioning of My Brain (What Remains of It)

I am fortunate that the conscious, "thinking" portion of my brain survived the accident more or less intact. Similarly, my memory works about as well as it did before. I have occasional forgetful moments like we all do, yet by and large I remember things well. My wife, in fact, depends on me to remind her of things—which seems misplaced when you figure she's married to someone with a brain injury—but her faith must not be radically out of place since I mostly succeed.

The reverse side of my thinking brain performance is that most of the visible things that involve the brain are damaged. I shudder to think of the impression I must make with the wheelchair, sagging face, jerky movements, loud voice, poor speech, and poor hearing. I'm like a computer where the CPU and memory mostly work OK, but all the peripherals and input/output devices are defective. If you know me mostly from email I seem fine, but in-person it's clear there are serious issues.

All of the above notwithstanding, I definitely do have some mental deficits. These impacts may be subtle to most observers, but I certainly notice them. For instance, I can't make cogent oral points. I always feel a step slow. When my wife and I argue (yes, it happens, though rarely), she always wins. I've given up even trying.

The injuries have changed my perspective markedly. Before the accident, I had to make snap judgments about people based on a quick sample of outward characteristics. Now, I wonder if I missed some remarkable hidden qualities. Certainly, my own interior life is much richer than it appears from the outside.

I can only do one thing at a time and must think intently about everything in order to do it. Psychologists say that multitasking is a myth and that everyone simply switches focus rapidly between multiple actions. If so, the absence of the ability to juggle things quickly is certainly amplified with me. Maybe it was a myth, but I acutely miss my old ability to multitask.

Difficulty with multiple simultaneous activities is most obvious with balance. Most uninjured people instinctively move their limbs, trunk, and head to stay in balance. I must concentrate on my center of mass to position my body parts in a way that requires minimal support to prevent falling. Even so, I usually need to hold on.

Other examples of my inability to multitask include turning on a light switch, especially with my left hand. I have to focus on the motion of my arm and hand. I typically need to halt any other activity (including propelling my wheelchair) if I try to speak. I cannot move and do something at the same time.

One therapist clearly demonstrated this process a few years ago. She had me try to stand while assembling a simple preschool-level jigsaw puzzle. Though I could do each thing alone (that is, either standing or assembling the puzzle), trying to do the two actions simultaneously proved extremely difficult.

I still routinely work on my multitasking by reading while standing for a few minutes. My ability has improved some, yet I continue to struggle with doing more than a single task simultaneously.

A not-so-obvious piece of this is that I must stay concentrated until some action is completely finished. It took a while for me to realize that finishing an action requires conscious focus. We all tend to focus until the key part of an action is over, then just let things finish automatically. I can't do this anymore. A simple example is applying toothpaste to a toothbrush. Putting the cap back on is a trivial automatic activity for most, but I need to concentrate until the tube is back on the counter.

Another piece that has become a major obstacle since my accident is panic attacks. I have always had some claustrophobia (fear of confined spaces) and acrophobia (fear of heights), but since my brain injury these irrational fears have intensified dramatically.

The attacks must have something to do with the disruption

of my brain chemistry, since an SSRI medication seems to hold them at bay much of the time. (I also suffer from depression if not medicated, though avoiding panic episodes seems to need the drugs more keenly.) If I don't take enough of the drug, I have panic attacks. The attacks are a strange situation, because I consciously know I am fine (for instance, just sitting in a room), yet the attack continues anyway. It's terrifying. Without the drug, I can feel panicked just sitting within my own skin (not a good feeling).

One trigger for these attacks is feeling constricted by clothing. I know some autistic people have problems with tags in their clothing. This is not the same, but I can understand. In contrast, an antidote seems to be feeling cold. Hence, I tend to underdress in the winter (one reason for wearing shorts all year) to help ward off these attacks. In warm weather when I'm wearing light clothing anyway, the attacks seem not to happen.

The problem is that SSRIs have side effects, notably sexual, so I try to minimize the dosage. Heavy doses of SSRIs can also make me feel emotionally numb, which has both advantages (mourning the death of my mother was easier) and disadvantages (losing emotional perspective when I write). Thus, I try to maintain myself at the edge. I try to take the minimum dose of medication that prevents panic attacks and use other behavioral measures as best I can.

The engineer in me has tried to sort out exactly what is going on with all these impacts, as if the big dent in my skull isn't a clear enough reason. I have wondered if many of the issues stem from delays in nerve transmission. I am aware, for instance, of the stuttering behavior of a remote arm (think *robot*) on trying to touch a hard surface due to transmission delays in its controls. My left leg does something similar. For another example, transmission delays would make balance much more difficult.

Obviously, the chemical nature of my brain is messed up. I don't have proper feeling on my left side. And some parts of my head (like audio on the right) simply do not function. Muscle weakness could result from the inability of nerves to get all the muscle fibers firing together. Coordination issues could result from a combination of transmission delays and muscle weakness.

None of this speculation really matters to improving my daily life. I just wonder.

A positive piece of the accident is that I am much more patient than I used to be. Spending hours lying in a hospital bed staring at the ceiling will do that. Imagine doing that as the prototypical type A I was. No wonder I fell apart.

The contrast is evident in everyday life when I compare myself to my wife. Now, she seems frequently impatient (for example, in traffic). Previous to the accident, she always seemed the patient half of our marriage. She hasn't changed (though she would argue that she has so much more to do now that I'm disabled), so I must have. I am quite capable now of retreating into my mind to work out things (for instance, the plot line of some story), so delays are no longer bothersome.

Similarly, I feel much less stressed than I used to. I didn't realize how tense I always was until responsibility fell away from my shoulders. I always felt driven, busy, and impatient. I would lose my temper over many things, including those like the weather that no one controls.

Now, I am more accepting when things don't go the way I'd like. I certainly recognize I have less control than I used to have, but it's not just suppressing my frustrations. I truly don't worry about things as much. Why? Perhaps it's the way the world proceeded without a hiccup when I disappeared unexpectedly for months. Perhaps I've always been content to be a follower. Perhaps it's the fact that I have to concentrate on the present to do things and thus can't take time to think about other issues. Given how hard people pursue mindfulness, I take this as a benefit.

I have more recently begun to ramp up my daily goals for myself. I have found that the old adage "do it once, you're congratulated; do it twice, it becomes an expectation" holds true. While this nugget of wisdom can apply to family or friends, it also applies to me. No matter how much effort and planning go into achieving something, I feel tempted to treat it after the first time as an everyday thing. I have to remind myself frequently that functioning in any way should not be taken for granted.

Communication

I no longer rely on a letter board to communicate. My text-to-speech app on my tablet sits unused. Verbal interaction remains challenging, but I can do it most of the time. As I said earlier, speaking clearly requires lots of concentration, but it is a much better situation than it once was.

When I verbally communicate (speaking and listening), something interesting happens. I experience a delay between hearing something spoken and registering its meaning. The same thing happens when I speak, a delay between forming the intent to speak and actual sound coming out. Though I've tried to understand it, like daily variations in my balance, I don't have a definitive answer. Perhaps there is a communication delay between the two halves of my brain. Regardless of the cause, the issue certainly slows down any conversation.

Much of my communication now goes by email. This route ensures that my garbled speech does not get in the way. I know this tactic can be frustrating for others sometimes, yet it prevents misunderstandings.

My writing by hand is poor. Attempting to write points out clearly how much coordination I have lost on the right side. Fortunately I was right-handed anyway. My left hand now would be even more hopeless. If I go very slowly, the words are mostly legible. I try to form the letters the same way I always have (my handwriting used to be strong), yet the result is not good.

I used to be a touch typist, able to work at the keyboard without looking. I was not incredibly fast or accurate, but the ability to type certainly helped in my work. That ability is gone, and I now have to type with one finger (right index) while staring at the keys. It's far slower but manageable. In addition, I rarely needed a spell-checker before (I usually found it annoying and turned it off), but now this aid has become very handy since mistakes happen frequently.

Reading is slower than it used to be yet still is a source of pleasure. With my nystagmus in the left eye, I frequently lose my place, especially when moving across the page to the next line. Moving line by line with a bookmark helps (credit my wife for that idea). Reading off a laptop screen at close range seems OK, but using a desktop monitor (even with enlarged type) is a struggle. Things move around too much.

I don't use a phone. In an emergency, I can use one, but in everyday life it has no place. Unthinkable as it might be for some, I have no cell phone.

A funny story. At work one day after being hurt, the desk phone rang, and I picked up the receiver and placed it against my right ear, just as I always did before the accident. Of course, the right ear is my deaf ear, so I heard nothing. It took me a few seconds to realize what was happening and to switch to my left ear.

I have set all the TVs in the house to use closed captioning. This step allows me to turn off the sound (or keep it low when I'm not alone in the room). I have tried using headphones so that loud sound won't impose on others, but then I struggle to make out conversation. I suspect that not only is my remaining hearing poor, my ability to decode words has been reduced. Slightly less than perfect audio and video synchronization may also contribute, since I naturally read lips to some extent.

Similarly, I can only make out fragments of speech (maybe one word in fifty) in a movie theater, a play, or other group event. Echoes—which occur almost everywhere in larger settings—seem to elude me. If a movie has subtitles, I am fine. Otherwise, I miss the dialog (which sometimes doesn't matter). It is strange to be at a movie or other public venue and see everyone else laughing when a humorous line passes, having no idea what has been said.

Eating and Drinking

Ingesting food and drink is vital to a living human. It's also one of the great joys in life. I can scarcely imagine going without consuming things by mouth for a whole year, though somehow I did. The fact that using a G-tube became routine shows just how much I adapted.

Today, I eat and drink by mouth and have no G-tube. I need to stay conscious of what I am doing, but otherwise have no hard restrictions. I avoid things that require a lot of chewing (like most steaks) since I have trouble with them. Small pieces and ground meat are not a problem. I also avoid things like spaghetti and linguine, which I tend not to be able to eat with any modicum of decorum due to my face being numb. I eagerly eat other pasta, where I can spear it with a fork. Soups are a messy item.

With only one decent hand, I am also a bit limited at the table. I cannot use a knife to cut things. I can use the edge of a fork to break up larger pieces (for instance, chicken filets and many vegetables) since I require relatively small pieces for eating. Green salads are a little tricky, but I can usually manage. (I love leafy greens, so it's not a question of forcing something I don't like.)

My tastes have changed only modestly. I still dislike the same things (raisins, eggplant, excessive blue cheese). One thing that has changed is that I no longer over-salt everything as I did pre-accident. I still like salt, just don't demand that everything taste salty. I believe this change happened when I was off solid food for such a long time.

Washing things down proves a greater challenge than solid food. Liquids run fast (the enemy of people with swallowing problems) and are harder to control. As long as I take small sips and concentrate, things tend to work out fine. It can take a long time to rehydrate when I'm exercising in warm weather, though I can do it given enough time.

I have had to give up grapefruit juice due to issues with my meds, but I consume orange juice, milk, and sports drinks just fine. I have always liked plain water (still or fizzy, chilled or not), so I manage to stay hydrated without trouble.

I should note that I often use a napkin holder (like used at a dentist) to form something like a bib with a napkin. It keeps my clothes neater. At first I felt self-conscious using it in restaurants, but now I am accustomed to it. It can't make me any more of a spectacle than I already am.

Speaking of restaurants, yes, I do eat out. I did not do so initially, but my wife loves to go out to dinner—we often used to go before I was hurt—so I have adapted.

The process of eating out is still somewhat more stressful for me than staying home, yet not nearly so much as in the beginning as a disabled person. I eat less and more slowly than I used to. The speed is typically not an issue since we are taking our time. I need to order purposefully (fileted seafood is usually good) to avoid issues associated with eating with only a single hand.

One problem that crops up both at home and away: I have trouble talking during meals. I'm not referring to speaking with my mouth full, which is always bad manners, but with simple conversation during a meal. In addition to requiring mental focus, speaking between swallows is physically difficult. The process is like asking my throat to switch between two modes: eating/swallowing and speaking. The solution is often to invite others to a meal, so my wife has someone to chat with.

Clothing

As I mentioned earlier, I wear shorts and a T-shirt essentially all year, with a sweatshirt when it is cool, to ease logistics and help ward off panic attacks. For things like PT, the attire seems practical as well.

When the occasion calls for something more dressy, I usually wear a polo shirt (short or long sleeves as dictated by the season). I have some athleisure pants when shorts are inappropriate. I still have a closet full of button-down shirts and ties that I can wear on special occasions.

Since I am sitting most of the time, I tend to wear oversized pants. The extra room in the waist and extra length fit better when seated. I don't use any of the adaptive clothing that is now available. I appreciate the idea, but I seem to manage OK with what I have.

I don some sort of footwear all the time. I propel my manual wheelchair in large part with my feet, so I need the traction.

To walk, I rely heavily on sensing my feet on the floor, so I need shoes with minimal padding. Most running shoes (what I most often wore pre-accident) have far too much cushion. Skateboarding shoes, especially the inexpensive kind, fall much closer to the mark in terms of a more direct connection to the floor. In hot weather, I wear sport sandals.

The only time when clothing can be an issue is at outdoor events in cooler weather. While I have no trouble getting from a car to inside a building even in winter wearing shorts, I have to wear something warmer for things like football games.

Chapter 8

Divestment

"Sometimes you need to clear away old things to make room for something new."

A psychologist told me that, probably trying to make me feel better about leaving something behind. Though true, this observation is not easy for me to accept.

I accumulated many things over my life before getting hurt as I had lots of interests. Many of these things became unusable after I became disabled, and I have said goodbye to them. For these items, it became somewhat emotional for me since I tend to form attachments to physical objects and feel committed to them. I try to remember that it doesn't have to be sad.

The first thing that went away was the mountain bike I crashed on. The bike survived the wreck pretty much unscathed (unlike me), but it quickly became clear I wouldn't ride it again, both because I physically couldn't and because of the unfortunate associations. My wife took the bike to a consignment sale at the same bike shop where I had bought it. Unbelievably, my helmet sustained no visible damage. As recommended, my wife tossed it anyway.

We also had to get rid of the tandem bicycle that my wife

and I toured on each year. The tandem was a recumbent (a recumbent tandem is a rare beast), and a handful to drive even unhurt, so there was no chance of still using it. The two of us had many great memories, but the bike went to a good home with a family with a handicapped child (so that the father could take the child on rides), so that eased the parting.

I still keep my old road and touring bikes. I don't have any hope of using them again, but their resale value is small (they were eleven and twenty-six years old at the time of my accident). Perhaps someday, I will find them a good place to go.

We had multiple boats. I had put the runabout in winter storage just before my accident. In fact, I had just pulled all the boats out of the water. The runabout proved relatively simple for my wife to dispatch: just have the people that stored it hold onto it and sell it on consignment. I loved that boat, but I would never be able to use it again.

We had two sailboats, the larger of which sat on a trailer in a garage at our house in town for the winter. I knew its days with us were numbered even before I became disabled. Stepping the mast each spring posed a challenging chore for me that would become more difficult to handle as I aged.

In addition, the craft had once capsized at its mooring in a storm and proved very difficult to right. Still, I had put a lot of work into the boat (I had recently refinished all the woodwork) so I had a lot of emotional ties to it. In the end, we sold it to some local people. The other, much smaller sailboat, a pedal-powered boat, the kayaks, and a canoe remained at the lake.

We kept my pickup truck for a few years since it made

hauling my trike possible. (My wife drove a small hybrid in those days.) After much debate, we traded both the truck and the hybrid when we bought a minivan. A minivan might seem like a big vehicle for a couple with no children at home and no grandchildren, but its low floor made loading my trike much easier for my wife.

Though I tried to learn to drive with my disability, I could not due to my weak vision. Surrendering my driver's license was another form of divestment.

You may be wondering what happened to our lake house, which we dearly loved. The place sat mostly unvisited for a couple years. I visited once after my injury, but it had lots of stairs, so the place was a poor match for me in my new state. I had designed it with a first-floor master suite, but stairs were required to get in from the parking area, and a long flight ran down to the dock. My wife hired someone to cut the grass and plow the snow (among the jobs I used to do there), but the house needed more care and a more consistent presence.

One winter a couple years into my disability, my wife came to me with a curiously large electric bill for the cottage. We were both mystified since the building was heated with propane. Long story short, a pipe had burst in the master bath. The excessive electrical draw ended up being from the well pump running constantly for weeks. The entire place had flooded, and water was everywhere. This would not have happened before my accident, when I used to go out to the cottage a couple times a week throughout the year. The place was fully winterized, and we used to cross-country ski on the lake.

The building had to be mostly gutted, though insurance

covered most of the reconstruction. In reality, the water damage proved a blessing in disguise, since it took further thought out of our hands. In addition to wrecked furniture, the water destroyed all my woodworking gear, my diving and snorkeling equipment, and numerous other things I'd never use again. After the rebuild and refurnishing, my wife put the cottage on the market as a furnished second home.

We sold the place to a local widower with young kids who hoped to use it for family gatherings. The pedal boat, my kayak, and the canoe went with it. The small sailboat had been sold as part of the flood cleanup. My wife retained her kayak in town.

Seeing the cottage go was sad, especially since I had built a number of things, but the place made no sense to keep. We have since spent a few days at the same lake—one of my wife's friends has a cottage there—and I remain on the lake association email list, though it's not the same without being able to fish and swim and sail.

I have also said goodbye to my guns. My brother and his family took them out to Wisconsin, where they still carry on the hunting and shooting traditions. It's possible that some guns remain (I had quite a collection), but if so they are locked in a gun cabinet (unloaded as always). Not only can I not reach them, I don't even know where a key is anymore.

I imagine the guns were taken away in part so that I couldn't hurt myself. No one needed to worry. If I seriously contemplated doing myself harm (which I haven't; see previous discussion), a firearm would be one of my last resorts, since I know that the event would only contribute to the stigma surrounding guns. My father always taught not only love but healthy respect and safe handling for weapons. Though he's gone, I wouldn't wish to disappoint him.

In this case, I saw no need to protest. My son and I had gone out target shooting once after my accident, but my vision proved too poor to make a trip to the range worthwhile ever again. I was not dangerous, just woefully inaccurate. If I had no legitimate use for firearms (target shooting and hunting had once been joys), I could see no point in keeping them.

Much of my other outdoor gear, such as my backpacking equipment, remains since it was stored in town. My son is an enthusiastic hiker, but he has all his own gear. Perhaps one of his friends will use my old equipment someday. My ski gear departed in one of the periodic purges (my wife is into decluttering).

Many of the yard tools have stayed, since someone needs to take care of the yard. The big gasoline-powered snowblower, which I'd had for a long time, got bartered away for some maple syrup. The trade made sense since the machine was much too big for my wife to handle. We got her a corded electric, though a plowing service does most of the snow clearing. My wife likes to mow the lawn (ours is small). The elderly gas mower finally died, and I got my wife, a new lightweight battery-operated mower that she loves.

I retain my hand tools. I rarely use them, but occasionally they help. Most of my power tools perished in the flood at the lake. The few that remain will probably go to my son at some point.

So what has replaced all these things? Obviously, my wheelchairs come to mind. I now ride a recumbent trike, which I love. I have acquired an extensive array of baking gear and ingredients. I adapted most of my existing gym equipment, though I have bought a few things. And I have transitioned almost exclusively to a laptop computer.

Chapter 9

On Faith

K *yrie eleison.*
I have known since I was a kid that the Latin words meant "Lord have mercy," but I never truly understood them viscerally until I was hurt. Lying in the hospital brought their beseeching meaning home in a very personal way. As low as I was then, I shudder to think that there may be an even deeper layer of understanding, though I'm sure there is.

I debated whether to have a chapter on religious faith. I expect some readers will be instantly repelled, either because they have no religious beliefs or because those beliefs are so central to their life that they can't imagine I could go this far without mentioning my own. For me, these beliefs are very important, yet very private.

As a compromise (something bound to make no one happy), I have chosen to limit my remarks on this subject to this chapter. This tactic is not a reflection of the importance of these beliefs in my life but a recognition that everyone does not share them, be their own different or nonexistent. This chapter can be skipped by those who wish to do so.

"On Faith" seems an appropriate title for this chapter. I

read somewhere that evangelicals dislike the word *religion*, and I think I understand why. Religion is a human construct, hence flawed. Faith is personal. Faith can be experienced and relied on by anyone. *Belief* is another good word.

I also don't wish to foment an argument with nonbelievers. Either one believes, or one doesn't. At its most basic, one either has a belief in a supreme being or one doesn't. If one doesn't believe, I can certainly understand how silly many religious rituals appear.

Nothing anyone can say proves or disproves the existence of a deity. Both religious advocates and atheists can readily point to historical examples where religion inspired great works or terrible mayhem, depending on the case. Like all human institutions, organized religion has its problematic issues, but when practiced appropriately, I argue it can enable selfless deeds that can elevate us all.

All of that said, I am a practicing Catholic (speaking of a complex legacy). Does that mean I think that any other faith tradition is not inspired? No. The idea may be heretical, but I think that elements of many religions have merit. I am not naive enough to think that my upbringing in a Catholic family had no influence. If I had been raised in the Islamic tradition, who knows the outcome. Similarly, I don't think that faith traditions are the sole way to view ethical and moral issues. One can be a very ethical and moral atheist.

Do I buy all the beliefs espoused by the Catholic church? Yes. I do not think it is wise to flout the dogma that has been handed down for hundreds of years. People much smarter and more educated than me have developed a self-consistent (or at least nominally self-consistent) program of beliefs. Picking and choosing those tenets that match one's own feelings is not necessarily self-consistent. At the same time, I understand that things evolve, sometimes in response to advocacy, so one needs to think for oneself, not just blindly follow old rules. Making those judgments on what to keep or change is central to the challenge of being part of a large church.

I won't debate all the hot-button issues here. In most cases, the problems are complex and not amenable to simple solutions.

Finally, as a scientifically trained individual, I can understand all the practical explanations for what some believe are religious phenomena. Take the case of near-death experiences. Though I stopped breathing and nearly died following my accident, I did not have the usual near-death experience described by many. Maybe I wasn't close enough to death. I am familiar with the narrowing visual field caused by hypoxia. Perhaps that is what so many experience.

Take the Trinity as another example more specific to my religion. I accept wave-particle duality in looking at subatomic particles, though I don't fully understand it. (Does anyone?) Although it's different, I can also accept the Trinity as being multiple manifestations of a single thing.

I don't believe in a literal interpretation of Scripture. Inspired, yes; literal, no. For example, I do think the earth is billions of years old. Maybe it isn't that ancient, and God is tricking all the scientists into thinking it's old by creating so much evidence of great age, but that's not my thinking.

Religious faith is not necessary to explain observed phenomena, though neither is it ruled out. There are new mysteries each time we look deeper. For instance, scientists have often defined what separates humans from other animals (use of tools is one old but not-obscure case). Yet each time something is identified as uniquely human, researchers then find this trait in another species. Thus, we can't even point to something specific that makes humans unique, yet we believe we are.

The role of faith in my recovery from injury has been paramount. It has given me perspective and a will to persevere.

Initially in DHMC, I was too stunned and sedated to think about faith. The stunned piece mostly continued at Spaulding. I remember a chapel there, but I did not connect to it. Looking back, I initially thought the reason for my avoidance of religion was that I felt angry at God. Mad about losing so much. Mad about the suffering I was enduring.

On further reflection since then (what some might consider revisionism), my guess is that I was too absorbed by simply trying to survive to think further. One would hope that I would rely on belief more fully in that extremity. That I didn't is perhaps a sign that my faith in God isn't deep enough.

One area where faith did help me in those early months was in the dismissal of suicide as an option. I believed (still do) that God brought me into this world, and I had no right to change anything so fundamental. If I was meant not to survive, there were ample opportunities for me to go away, if that was God's will. I certainly prayed to die, but I took no other action.

Matters changed in my long stay at Crotched Mountain. I still did not attend any formal religious gatherings, except one ecumenical service at Easter, but I had more time to think. I came to the conclusion that my accident was not the work of God. Though I certainly felt deserving of suffering (the Catholic in me comes through), the God I believe in does not punish people that way. My accident was not mandated by God.

At the same time, I can't help thinking that the accident was somehow meant to happen. A few minutes longer without a rescue team, and I would have stopped breathing, lying there in the woods. A few inches to one side, and I might have missed the rock with my head completely and not fractured my skull. So many contingencies were required to line up.

I've never figured out how I threaded the complex and narrow passage to where I am now. It remains mysterious to me. All I know is that if my survival and recovery can be viewed as a testament to God, the struggle to move forward will be justified. I survived for a reason, though I am not smart enough to figure out the reason.

Since returning home, I have returned to attending Mass regularly. My wife is not Catholic, so it is extra effort on her part to make sure I'm there. Strangers have wheeled me to Communion in a manual wheelchair. I cannot understand the spoken prayers for the most part, but it hardly matters since I know them so well. What does matter is that God knows I'm there, trying.

I do not pray to be restored to an able body, as nice as that would be. Rather, I pray to be up to the challenges ahead.

Despite my faith, I do still fear death, though not as starkly as I would otherwise. When I do go, I expect to see loved ones who are deceased, like my mother and father. That about completes my vision of an afterlife. It's too complicated for me to understand in any greater depth.

Could I be wrong about this whole religious faith thing? Certainly. I know that it may just be a folly and that others may have the last laugh at my expense. Perhaps the human animal needs something to cope with the mysteries of the natural world, the vagaries of chance, and the seeming permanence of death. (As a coping mechanism alone, does that sound so bad?) Belief must confer some evolutionary advantage to have appeared in so many forms.

Perhaps. But I believe there's a consciousness behind it all. My view of structured religion may be more critical since I was injured, but my belief in a supreme being is greater.

Chapter 10

Mobility

"There is more to life than a car."
My father said something like this when I was a teen and gaga about cars. At that time, my world revolved around cars, be they fast or simply great-looking. He viewed them more as necessary evils, things we needed for living life. Looking back, he was more right than wrong.

Manual Wheelchairs

The manual wheelchair has been the first and foremost way that I get around since being hurt. I currently have three manual chairs: one that I use most often inside the house on the main level; an inexpensive chair on the lower level when I have to descend indoors; and an outdoor chair that I use outside and on excursions.

Chairs are highly personal things. They become almost part of you. I will describe my choices with the stipulation that these things work for me at this phase of my life, certainly not for everyone. I am fortunate to retain limited use of my legs so that transfers are simpler, and I don't need to spend all my waking hours in the chair.

First, I use a lightweight folding chair with an aluminum frame. I know that titanium chairs are lighter (though appreciably more expensive) and that rigid chairs have many advantages, but these folding aluminum chairs have served me well. Next, I rely on hard non-pneumatic wheels. I know lighter wheels with pneumatic tires would perform better, but the maintenance aspect is too daunting given that I'd mostly need to do it myself (my wife is not mechanical).

As far as personal preferences, I use adjustable-height armrests that pivot out of the way. I have long arms and find standard-height armrests too high, so I leave the adjustable-height armrests at their lowest setting. I take advantage of the pivoting armrests to transfer. I didn't do so initially but have come to rely on it.

On cushions, I use a foam cushion with a minimal anatomic shape. For a long time (too long), I put up with a slippery air-permeable cushion cover on my inside chair. When I got my now-outside chair, it came with an impermeable cushion (different brand) that wasn't nearly as slippery. To save money, before buying a whole new cushion, I tried an impermeable cover on the inside chair. Though it looks shiny and slippery, this new cover represents a huge improvement. I don't tend to slide out of this chair anymore. The lesson in all of this is to insist on the cushion one needs since it makes a big difference.

I don't use leg rests on any of my wheelchairs except on rare occasions. I rely too much on my legs to propel me. Since my issues are mainly on my left side, my left arm can't do much on the handrim and requires intense focus to do what little it can. Using the handrims to move only works in confined spaces indoors. While I sometimes use my hands on the rims, it is merely a fine-tuning supplement to the propulsion provided by my legs, principally the right leg. If someone is pushing me a long distance, I will use leg rests so that I don't need to hold up my legs for a long time.

I had hoped that a lever drive for my wheelchair would enable me to be more independent outside. I procured a lever drive that was integrated into a set of new wheels. I practiced in the dead-end street in front of our house (where a neighbor mildly hit me when backing her car, but that's another story). Yet, though the levers helped some, they could not help me overcome my left-right strength imbalance. In addition, the lever drive increased the weight of the chair, making it more difficult to load in a car. Finally, the levers contributed to a small increase in width that made passing through doorways trickier. Now, I don't use the levers.

A result of using my feet so much is that I have little to no tolerance for throw rugs. I can sometimes tolerate large area rugs as long as they are thin, but I tend to pull throw rugs into tangles with my feet. The difficulty is that my wife adores rugs and wants to use them broadly. We compromise by having rugs only in locations I don't travel. (I have no doubt that rugs will immediately appear throughout the house when I am no longer on the scene.)

On this same subject, I note that thick carpeting poses a huge problem. Most of our house has hard-surface floors, which makes getting around much easier. When we travel and stay in hotels, the carpet creates a huge problem. The thick pile may absorb sound and feel comfortable underfoot for the able-bodied, but the rolling resistance nearly incapacitates me.

I have mixed feelings on a positioning (or seat) belt on a wheelchair. I have belts on two of my three chairs today and only use them sporadically. Until I had a non-slippery cushion cover, a belt helped to keep me from sliding out of my indoor chair. Now that I have the correct cushion cover, I no longer need the belt, and it seems to mostly get in the way.

I often use partially fingered wheelchair gloves outside the house for a few reasons. Unlike for many people who use them, gloves aren't necessary to alleviate sore hands from excessive use, since I normally rely on my feet. Gloves do help in providing a better grip on the handrims and protect my hands from damage from the wheels. Gloves also provide some additional warmth, which is often helpful with my poor circulation.

Let me insert a word about chair setup. Many modern wheelchairs have extensive adjustability. My advice is to use that ability, since the adjustments can make a big difference. I have adjusted the center of balance partway on my chairs. For many users, putting most of their weight on the back (main or large) wheels not only makes a chair more maneuverable—and able to easily do wheelies—but can reduce the energy needed to move. Unfortunately, my balance is so poor that it's safer not to adjust the chair weight distribution further. I also use anti-tip wheels to prevent accidents.

I have an odd relationship with my wheelchairs. Though I resent having to use one, I also value them. My chairs make me independent. I don't need someone with me to use them. Also, a wheelchair is a very visible symbol of disability. While several of my issues are not casually observable, the wheelchair makes it obvious I have infirmities. At times, it seems to generate empathy and respect on the part of others.

Walkers and Other Mobility Aids

Since I have some use of my legs, I can use a walker, though only with close supervision. I have a rollator that I use mostly at PT. It is of the standard configuration and folds front to back. I have not tried the so-called Euro-style rollators that fold side to side. I doubt it would make a substantial difference. I once tried a rollator intended for Parkinson sufferers but didn't see much difference. I also have a conventional lightweight walker on the lower level of the house.

I will sometimes use a four-point cane at PT, but only with a therapist holding on. I have such a cane at home but rarely utilize it since I can't use it by myself and my wife is too petite to aid me. I rely heavily on sensing my balance through my feet, which is problematic at best.

I would be remiss if I didn't mention the parallel bars in my home gym. They allow me to work on walking alone.

I know I won't walk normally again, but I keep the training going as if I will. The attitude is "futility be damned." And all the effort is not totally futile. While my inner ear remains the same, I have trained my proprioception to play a bigger role. I would be the first to tell you my balance is still way off and it requires continuing practice, but I walk straighter and taller and place far less pressure on my hands these days. If nothing else, trying to walk is good exercise.

Power Mobility

I recently added a power wheelchair (power chair) for getting around town. Back when I was able-bodied, I never got the convertible sports car I wanted, so this feels like an approximation suited to my current abilities.

I don't use the power chair in the house at this time. I have enough problems hitting things in a manual chair. I can only imagine the damage I'd do with a power chair. Since we don't have a wheelchair van or a decent van ramp, I use the power chair only to travel from home. Fortunately, we live within walking (or power chair) distance of many things.

The power chair enables me to run errands in town with my wife or go to theaters, the grocery store, and the like. She still needs to go most places because of my limited vision and hearing. We can also go out to restaurants (within walking distance and in good weather) without requiring her to muscle me along. One quickly learns the condition of the sidewalks this way.

While they may seem simple, power chairs can require lots of concentration to drive, at least for me. Not only must one keep the chair from falling off the edge of the sidewalk, one must constantly be looking at the imperfections of the pavement coming up. I frequently practice driving, which seems a good excuse for getting outdoors as well.

I occasionally use the power chair on sidewalks in near darkness. For this, I have mounted a flashing rear light (from cycling) and wear a headlamp. Since my vision is limited, I don't do this often.

Of course, with batteries vulnerable to freezing, my power chair must be parked indoors during the winter. This limitation is no great hardship since the chair becomes too cold and exposed to ride in harsh weather anyway.

At four miles per hour, the power chair may not be fast, but it does give me back some sense of open-air motoring.

Electric Scooters

I have used an electric scooter at an outdoor fair. While it is fine for getting around, in close quarters—like a bathroom—it is unworkable. Scooters may be great for some, but the power chair is a better match to me since I can't walk at all.

Automobiles

I don't drive. I made an attempt to learn with some adaptive driving instructors, but my vision was too poor. I do fairly well in a static vision test where nothing is moving. My depth perception is not great with only one serviceable eye (as I've frequently proved by spilling liquids when trying to pour), but I seem to manage well enough.

My real downfall is when things start moving. My nystagmus in my working left eye makes it very hard to focus on moving objects. I seem to do adequately—but just adequately—until about twenty miles per hour. Beyond that speed I can't keep up. Since traffic moves at more than twenty miles per hour most of the time, I am better off not driving.

Since I can stand holding onto something, I can transfer to and ride in an unmodified vehicle, ours or one belonging to someone else. That fact tremendously increases flexibility since a wheelchair van is not required. I typically need to take the front passenger seat in a vehicle.

Since my wife is not always available, we have sometimes hired a driver. A very nice retired lady took me to work and PT for several years.

For vehicles, we now have an unmodified minivan, though previously we had a compact hybrid and my prior pickup truck. One may ask why a couple with no children at home and no grandchildren needs a minivan. The question disappears when one sees my trike loaded in without folding or disassembly. While our van now has handicap license plates, I still have a placard for use in other vehicles.

I am not a great navigator. I have trouble reading signs while we are driving. My overall sense of direction, which used to be uncanny, remains partly intact and helps occasionally.

Now that my wife is solely responsible for driving, our road trips are shorter and less frequent than previously. Bathroom breaks must be planned on road trips. Though I can manage in a minimal ADA restroom, some are much better than others. Traveling enough, one learns where the good bathroom facilities are. New destinations are always an adventure.

Air Travel

Traveling by air is doable but not easy. Air travel with a G-tube used to be similar with the additional caveat that we had to tote all my food, which significantly limited me.

The first step in air travel begins at reservation time. I look for direct flights. My one experience as a disabled person with making connections was not good, even with a wife who could push me to a new gate.

I have flown as far domestically as the Northeast to the Southwest in the continental US. I don't know if I could manage a trip to Europe or another overseas destination.

We take a bus from our town to a major airport, which has more direct flights. The bus has a wheelchair lift, which makes the trip straightforward. I say "we" since I always travel with a companion, usually my wife. Even if I managed to get around OK, my lack of vision and hearing make traveling alone impossible.

The trip from the curb to check-in remains fraught. My traveling companion must handle the luggage, so I do what I can to get to check-in on my own. Once free of the luggage (we always have to check bags), the process becomes easier, since I can be pushed.

In an airport, I am next to useless. I have trouble seeing the flight boards. I can't parse audio announcements. I used to fly regularly for my job, so I know many airports and quickly orient to strange places. That is my only advantage. In general, it's best to consider me akin to a companion animal.

Security screening is always a minor adventure. Many airports have a wheelchair shortcut that takes me to the head of the line, but it is still slow. At the screening portal I usually suffer a long delay while an extra security officer is found. Some people can get up from their wheelchair and walk through the portal. I cannot. It is necessary to find that spare officer to take me through a bypass. Once through the bypass, my chair and I are subject to a pat-down search. Some of the searches are very thorough (wearing shorts helps expedite this search), others less so. Frequently, I get a newly hired officer so that the correct search procedure is learned. Since my hearing deficit is not visible, I often have trouble interpreting the officer's oral instructions in what is usually a noisy environment. The extended search process negates any time I save by speeding through the special wheelchair queue.

At the gate, my companion always checks in at the desk. My wheelchair is typically given a gate check tag. Though everyone is nice, sitting there in my chair with a tag attached makes me feel like a piece of luggage. We are usually given seats near the front of the plane.

I find the boarding and exiting of the plane itself not a bad chore. Attendants typically help me into an airplane aisle wheelchair (very narrow) at the bottom of the jetway, then maneuver me aboard. Getting off is just the reverse. One important note, however, is that I'm often first on/last off the plane. Any advantage I might gain by early boarding is more than offset by being unloaded late. The cleaning crew members are often mostly finished by the time I exit. My own chair rides below as gate-checked baggage.

A last consideration looms large. Most aircraft and buses don't have accessible restrooms, so preparation for a trip involves fasting and dehydrating so I won't need to use a toilet. Airports usually have well-equipped accessible bathrooms, so I have to plan any eating and drinking around stops at those places. The simplest approach is often going without anything to eat or drink until I reach my destination.

Chapter 11

Vocations and Avocations

"**I**f I had half a brain."

I used to utter that expression when I did something dumb. Now that I literally have half a brain—whether exactly half or some other fraction—I have a ready excuse. Unfortunately, I find I need an excuse for doing dumb things too often.

I've always liked being busy, whether it's my job or hobbies. That hasn't changed. I still try to fill my days productively.

Work

My career as an R&D engineer largely ended in the crash. I had been doing the job successfully for over twenty years at that point. One might think that I could still function adequately since the thinking part of my brain remained largely intact. One would be wrong.

After two years on medical leave, I returned to work part time, a couple afternoons a week. My easy exhaustion precluded me from working more hours. My hearing, speech, and vision difficulties made communicating with coworkers difficult, more than I expected. I had a few panic attacks when I didn't police my thoughts carefully enough.

I was, of course, no longer the president or an owner of the company by the time I returned. Operations at the firm had moved on in the time I was away, as they had to do. I didn't work for the money (I was on disability) but to try to be useful.

As a disabled person, I mostly did marketing pieces for the company, which I had done since long before the accident. Whereas before getting hurt these pieces constituted only a minor part of my overall workload, now they were the main focus.

With effort, I could use a computer. I got a large-print keyboard and set the magnification up on my big-screen monitor. Even with those compensations, reading things on-screen (where my nystagmus made them jerk around) and writing messages proved a chore.

Email became the best means of communicating with me. Occasionally, I advised some of my colleagues on their projects. People went out of their way to be nice. The company set up a computer at my house so that I could easily work from home on days I couldn't come in. I got a few requests to help on sales efforts, supporting proposals and the like. I did some corporate history work. In short, the company and I tried many things to see if there was a perfect niche for me.

After over four years and dwindling roles, I fully retired. I felt resigned to this step. I could tell that I wasn't delivering at my old level. If positions were reversed, I knew that I wouldn't have tried further if I were the one of the managers overseeing my work. At that point, I no longer was sad to go. I had tried.

I gave lots of notice before leaving on this occasion. My wife thinks the company would probably have let me continue for a long time, but I knew that eventually someone would tap me on the shoulder and say "it's time." We had some nice retirement celebrations (at least I didn't wait until all my old colleagues had gone).

After retiring, I served for a while in on-call status, which meant I retired but remained available if needed. The need for me was negligible, as anticipated, so I terminated that status. In the unlikely case that I am needed, the company knows how to reach me.

The firm did me a final honor by naming a new conference room after me. Since the company only had two such named conference rooms in its over five-five-year history, it was an extremely humbling gesture.

Writing

The focus of my work life now centers on writing, which I have time to do in retirement. I had begun even before I went back to the office. At first, I pursued it as a lark, something I always wanted to do. Now, I'm more serious. I always knew I would need a second career when I retired. Writing fits this need.

Aside from this book you're reading, I focus on fiction. That seems strange, since I read mostly nonfiction (history, to be more precise). Maybe I had my fill of writing nonfiction in my professional work. Maybe I have turned to fiction since it means less research—though not none. A psychotherapist encouraged my fiction bent as an outlet for creativity. I read a lot of fiction as a young person, growing up and in college.

I even did a lot of writing. That habit got put on the shelf for decades as I pursued my career in engineering.

Thus far, I have written six novels and almost a dozen short stories. Only a couple of the short stories have been published. Four of the novels are in a series. Nobody told me (perhaps I should have gotten some instruction) that writing a series of novels forms a trap, since one depends on the first book in the series to set a good tone. The first in my series was pretty dreadful, since I had just started writing. That novel has improved with new drafts, but it has taken a lot of effort, and I'm not finished, though the most recent revisions seem a major improvement to me. I have ideas for a few more novels.

The short stories have evolved better. The first story I wrote in just a couple days after being asked by a medical student we were hosting for dinner. The publishing of that story felt positive, though I felt like I had an in. The second thing I published seemed like a stronger affirmation since I had no connection to the literary magazine and it was the only fiction story published in that annual edition of the journal, beating out over one hundred rivals.

I have to guard against getting too serious. I don't seek a return to stress. Right now, writing remains fun and not a formal job. I need to keep it that way.

Culinary Pursuits

Beyond writing, my big avocation now is baking. I have always liked to cook, even back in the long-ago days in college when I made very limited stuff. I can't stand at the stove for very long now, and my knife skills (never great) are especially weak due to using mostly one hand and a semi-coordinated one at that. Baking, as I practice it, is less time-critical and more tolerant of my flaws.

I began to bake as a disabled person when my old bread machine died and we bought a new, fancy one. Long ago, I had baked a few things like bread, pretzels, focaccia, and pizza crust with the old machine. With the new machine, I began baking bread. In fact, since we got this machine over nine years ago, I have made all of our bread. After a few months of baking bread, I moved on to desserts. At present, I bake a dessert about once a week and keep us supplied not only with several types of bread and rolls but also cakes, pies, cookies, breakfast cereal, pizza, focaccia, pretzels, bagels, and energy bars.

A couple years ago, I tried using the ice cream maker that my stepson had left behind when he moved out. Now, along with the other desserts, I make homemade ice cream for us, too.

I also do a little cooking, mostly in the slow cooker. Again, the pace matches my glacial style. It takes me a long time to cut up ingredients, but the slow cooker is forgiving. In addition to traditional slow cooker items, I have adapted some other recipes. I usually cook one evening a week, and we can usually get at least two meals out of what I produce.

I have experimented on occasion. While many experiments are successful, I've had a few memorable duds. One St. Patrick's Day, I attempted to corn my own brisket. The result was far too salty despite rinsing the corned brisket with fresh water a few times. After that experience, I now focus on making Irish brown bread for the holiday, which turns out great.

These days, my culinary work is my contribution to the family. I can no longer mow the lawn, clear the snow, grill out, or maintain most mechanical things, but I can help in this way. Credit my wife with helping (I sometimes struggle to manage the oven with one hand) and doing the dishes (one task I know she wishes I could still manage). We often team up. Few of my wife's friends are into baking, so she sometimes shares things with them. As I like to say, "I haven't poisoned anyone yet." My wife is the superior cook, and likes working in the kitchen in moderate doses, but she tolerates and encourages me.

I should note that working in the kitchen exhausts me. One wouldn't think that doing something while sitting could be so tiring. It can be tempting to say "oh, I've made that before," but familiarity doesn't erase the energy demands on me. I get just as tired.

Chapter 12

Exercise and Recreation

"**Y**ou ought to have your head examined."

That's the (eminently reasonable) comment that some people make when they hear I am back cycling. To that remark, I say "I have" and pedal away.

I have always been a devotee of exercise and outdoor sports. As an able-bodied person, I did many things. I might not have been great at any one of them, but the sheer variety was impressive.

With the wheelchair and gimpy left side, not to mention lack of balance, days in the woods or on the water have been curtailed. I know they make all sorts of aids to allow disabled people to continue activities in the outdoors, but I now limit myself to a few because of the extra effort and expense involved.

Cycling

My primary sport has always been cycling. The combination of the mechanical and athletic has always meshed with me. I never competed (far from good enough), but I love it. I no longer ride off-road—which was not a large part of my activity anyway—but I immediately returned to road cycling.

My left leg is weak, yet I still pedal with it. The left leg is more than just along for the ride, but barely. My weak vision works well enough at the low speeds of cycling (especially *my* slow speeds) to permit me on the road. Plus, I pose much less a danger to others from my limited eyesight than I would driving a car. The use of a three-wheeled recumbent addresses my balance issues.

As I wrote earlier, I initially started with a delta trike (two wheels in back). Though the trike was fun and easy to mount, the riding height made it prone to capsizing for a balance-lacking person like me. (The configuration might be ideal for others.) A tadpole trike (two wheels in front) that was much lower to the ground worked better for me. Tipping over in the tadpole is still possible but much harder to do. To deal with the low seat, I use a car door or a grab bar in the garage to lower myself into the position.

After a couple years on my first tadpole, I bought a different one. I shipped my original tadpole to my brother's house in Wisconsin since we tend to ride a lot when I visit. The newer tadpole has full suspension and other goodies. I had them build it up with all shifting in my right hand but braking on both sides. My left hand struggled with shifting on my first tadpole yet seems to manage braking OK.

All my day rides are significantly shorter than they used to be. A long ride for me now is twenty to thirty miles. I go as far as fifty miles in some one-day events, but those occasions are special, and very draining. My wife gets me out two to three times a week in season. She rides behind me on a conventional road bike to help make me more visible to cars because I am so low to the ground. I also use a flag and flashing lights, front and rear. She must be extremely patient.

My routes are nearly entirely on quiet country roads or highways with bike lanes. We have very few paved trails nearby, though we have occasionally taken trips to places with paved trails. Once in a great while, I will ride on an unpaved trail, but the shaking of the rougher surface makes my nystagmus nearly intolerable.

I ride at a decent pace (still much slower than in pre-accident days) downhill and on the flats but am extremely slow on climbs, of which there are plenty in northern New England. I understand that the same uphill speed issues apply with handcycles.

A simple rule of thumb is to divide my pre-injury abilities by two. I mostly still ride roughly the same amount of time, but my speed and distance traveled is down by about half.

My wife and I used to tour together riding a recumbent tandem before I was hurt. Nothing like that happens now, though for six years we did a three-day hundred-mile ride for the disabled in the White Mountains. About three days straight is all I can manage, especially with all the climbing. I know it's best not to try to ride at the limit all the time, but my weak performance on uphills makes it impossible not to, assuming I want the ride to end in a reasonable time. (I had trouble going easy even when I was able-bodied.)

My brother and his family also like to ride, so we usually get together a couple times a year to do some cycling.

I don't need any special equipment, other than my trike, to ride. My prior cycling jerseys still work fine, though I have a few new garments, too. I use compression shorts designed for runners. Almost any short would do, but I like these because they are similar to snug cycling shorts (though usually cheaper) without the padding.

Since I can no longer wear contact lenses, I have retired my interchangeable-lens sunglasses for prescription photochromic glasses with plenty of coverage to keep out the wind (and bugs, gravel, and the like). I still utilize the same pedals and cycling shoes with recessed cleats that I formerly used for touring. Of course I wear a helmet, now with a flashing light I use on dim days.

One might think that as slow as I am on ascents, I make up for it downhill. Unfortunately, no. I no longer let it all hang out when the pavement turns down. Where I used to go forty-five-plus miles per hour regularly, I try to keep it to about twenty-five miles per hour or less now, even when it means laying on the brakes.

In perfect conditions (bright sun, great pavement I know well, wide paved shoulder or quiet road) I can go at twenty-five miles per hour or a little faster, but anything less than perfect slows me down. For example, sun dappling through the trees may look nice, but it disrupts my limited vision. That close to the ground, descending feels frightening enough at twenty-five.

The trike will certainly go faster than twenty-five miles per hour in many downhill situations, but I have to hold it back. Not only is my vision limited, my hands are not so steady anymore, and trikes handle quickly. I have a persistent dread of losing control at speed and rolling the trike. The outcome would not be pretty.

I would be remiss if I didn't mention that cycling is also mentally demanding for me. I must concentrate to keep the trike on the road lest I wander into a ditch or traffic. Focus is also needed to maintain pedaling. The situation has improved a bit over time, but I still need to consciously command my left leg to pedal on each stroke. The result is that I'm not a particularly social rider, since I can't talk and steer or pedal simultaneously.

Another impact on cycling I did not expect: refueling. Eating and drinking at rest stops requires much more time than formerly. I consume slowly while stopped. I cannot drink while moving, and things take time even when I halt. On shorter rides, this doesn't pose a problem since I can simply rehydrate and (if needed) replenish food when I get back home. The impact is felt on longer rides. The only solution I've found is patience.

I don't know if my injuries have affected my cardiovascular system. I wouldn't be surprised if they have, since most other body systems have been impacted by my TBI. I still endure the same struggles we all do when pushing myself athletically with burning muscles, laboring heart, and heavy breathing. At the same time, I still feel the intensely pleasurable rush of endorphins after a spirited ride ends. My struggles in endurance sports—before the accident, running was always hard as well—may be partially due to low iron levels. I once had a doctor refer to me as borderline anemic.

I'm still learning about recovery. At present, my thinking is that my right leg and most of my body bounce back from hard efforts in a day or two (like they used to in pre-accident days). My left leg takes a couple days longer. Since I rely most heavily on my right leg, additional cycling is within reason after a few days. For balance and walking where both legs must perform at the height of their reduced abilities, acceptable behavior (by my low standards) requires substantially more rest. At least that is my current thinking.

PT

Though some might view physical therapy as something else, I use it as a key part of my exercise routine.

The therapist has me walk with my rollator (holding on loosely) and sometimes with a cane (much more supportive). I can balance well enough (with concentration) to stand on my own for a short time. This ability can be deceiving. I have toppled over twice when a therapist didn't watch me carefully enough. In addition to walking, the therapists have me do other exercises for my legs and balance.

Beyond the lower body work, I also do some upper body and occupational therapy work from my chair at PT. As with walking, the changes are subtle.

I end each PT appointment with an extended session on a recumbent stepper. On this machine, the action of my legs (it works my arms as well) is similar to cycling. With the stepper's computer monitoring my performance, it provides an objective measure of my status. Thus far, my numbers are slowly but steadily improving.

I have learned something from each physical therapist I've had. I don't know if the longevity with one therapist is typical or not, but I worked with one woman for over five years. Though there are many commonalities, each therapist has some nuances in approach. I pay attention and have picked up a host of things to practice.

Weightlifting

I have enjoyed weightlifting on my own for decades. Really. I enjoy it. While many consider working with a pile of cast iron without company a chore that is difficult to maintain over time, I relish it. Nowadays, I don't lift nearly as much weight as I used to, but I still work out regularly in my home gym.

I won't go into a detailed account of my workouts—everyone's needs are different—but I do recommend resistance training. I read somewhere once that a guy ran a gym that specialized in wheelchair-bound people, saying "being strong helps one in a wheelchair." I wholeheartedly agree. Being physically fit helps in navigating life in a chair.

Lifting weights provides more evidence that my brain is not working properly. In addition to the weakness on my left side and reduced coordination on my right, a few strange artifacts arise. For instance, my left toes curl when I squeeze my right hand.

I do dumbbell work, floor exercises (knee pads are needed), and a few things with a bar. I use some of my old equipment. I know there are specialized machines for those in wheelchairs. Those machines might be great, but I don't have any. I accomplish a great deal with a few inexpensive dumbbells, some of my old gear, and resistance bands.

Skiing

In winter, I do sit-down alpine skiing, which gets my wife and I out of the house typically once a week. A mountain near us has a great adaptive program. Near our home here in northern New England, skiing is very popular, and adaptive programs are not uncommon. Cross-country skiing seems out due to the weakness in my left arm. With my weak balance, I stick to a dual-ski alpine configuration.

For the first few years, I tried to use handheld outriggers when adaptive skiing, since that seemed like the objective of all the people I saw on TV. These outriggers were extremely challenging to use due to the weakness on my left and lack of balance. I did pretty well when the instructor was hands-on with the sled but crashed a lot on a tether. The crashes were at low speed—mostly tipping over—so the risk of injury was slight. Beyond the frustration, however, crashing frequently is exhausting.

A few seasons back, the instructors tried fixed outriggers that mount to the sled. These worked much better for me. I still fall over if I lean too much, but I seem to be able to stay upright much better and can tackle additional terrain, even on a tether.

A word on gear is appropriate. I don't own the sled (sit-ski); it is provided along with instructors by an adaptive sports organization. Mostly I can utilize regular skiwear. I use oversize ski pants (which fit better when sitting) and a bigger than normal jacket to help prevent panic attacks. On my hands, I have electrically heated mittens. Not only is my circulation poor on the left, I can't sense temperature. Before I got these, when I used conventional mittens, the only way I knew my left hand had become cold was if it began to drag on the snow (not good with a handheld outrigger). Now with the heated mitten, I still can't sense temperature on the left, but I can keep that hand more functional.

Other Stuff

Beyond cycling and skiing as a disabled person, I have gone kayaking once or twice each summer with an adaptive program. If I am in a single kayak (sometimes I am in a tandem), the instructors add some outriggers to the boat to ensure I don't turn over. I'm not sure the outriggers are necessary, but people want to play it safe.

In fact, the only time I've ended up in the water was one trip after I'd exited the kayak and was standing on a launch ramp. A volunteer didn't hold me tightly enough (as I said earlier, my balance can be deceiving), and I fell into the river. I was wearing a life jacket so I was fine.

My paddling is not terribly strong anymore due to the weak left arm, yet it is nice to be out on the water.

I no longer hike, camp, snorkel, sail, fish, or hunt. There is adaptive equipment for many of these activities, but time is limited, plus without a waterfront house there is less convenience to the watersports I used to enjoy. If any of those sports were a particular favorite, I know I could pursue them if I were focused enough. (Well, maybe not the snorkeling.)

Indoors, I spend time reading (mostly history) and working on puzzles. Same as ever, I have a number of websites I follow. I do watch some television, though I try to limit it.

I go to occasional concerts (my wife sings in a chorus that mostly performs classical masterworks). I cannot understand most dialog in a theater, though I can hear music to some degree.

I have not tried to attend any country music events (my musical passion in the last several years before my accident) with my damaged hearing. I try to listen to headphones or earbuds, but the music often sounds strange even when I set things to monaural. I still can hear music in my head (I have a great memory that way), even down to the specific cracks and pops from the old vinyl I once used. Unfortunately, most of these memories terminate sometime when I was in college (i.e., decades ago). Thus, inside my head, the soundtrack is often like a weird oldies station.

Though I've tried repeatedly, I cannot play the trumpet anymore. I had played the horn since I was a young kid. I played in a classic R&B band as an adult. The problems are multifold, but the insurmountable one is that half my facial muscles are immobilized, preventing me from forming a working embouchure. Playing the horn would be excellent therapy in several dimensions if I could manage it.

Chapter 13

Miscellany

"Thank you."

The only proper response to the actions of others is "thank you."

In addition to the positive effects of gratitude on myself, a grateful attitude is nearly always appropriate. Even if someone doesn't do something exactly correctly or in accordance with my preferences, most people are trying to be helpful. They may not get it quite right since they are unused to the disabled or my disabilities in particular, but they are trying.

In the rare case where someone is apathetic or doesn't treat me with respect, I say "thank you" pretending I am being sarcastic. Note that I say "pretend." (Being a wiseass is not helpful.)

Being disabled has touched all facets of my life.

Alcohol

I have always liked a drink. Throughout my growing up, my parents drank regularly, though never to the point of intoxication. My grandfather on my father's side ran a liquor store, though he rarely drank himself. I shared my first beer with my father when I was sixteen, while on vacation. In her later years, my mother had one martini each evening before dinner. Thus, I grew up with frequent but not excessive use of alcohol. Everyone I knew modeled a healthy relationship with drinking.

I am thankful that I am still able to consume moderate quantities of alcohol. Now, one drink is about my limit. Even after one, I am less steady than usual. After a drink, I can barely manage transfers. Any more than one drink poses much too high a risk.

While in pre-accident days, I preferred red wine, nowadays I mostly drink beer. My intention with this choice is to stretch out each drink. The tradition now is that I tend to have a beer with dinner each night. Fortunately, there is an explosion of fine craft beers available now so quality is never an issue. If alcohol is not available, I'm fine with water.

Once a week, my wife and I have a cocktail. I make something, and she serves it. A number of recipes make up my cocktail repertoire now, and I like to try new things.

Why drink at all? I can walk away from the alcohol. In the first year after being hurt, I had to give up drinking alcohol entirely. I drink lots of water. Always have. I simply enjoy alcohol as one of the pleasures I can still indulge.

Fixing Things

Before my accident, I was moderately handy. I had given up working on cars (too complicated these days), but I did maintain our bikes and fix many things around the house. I had taken up woodworking. To my frustration, I can do almost none of those things since my accident. My son even has to change light bulbs when he visits.

I occasionally try to fix something simple despite the irritation it causes me and the excessive time it requires. The first issue is that I often take a long time to retrieve my tools. Though I mostly remember where the tools are, many times getting them entails a trip to the downstairs garage, which takes a long time even if the weather is good and I can go downstairs outside. Next, I have to get close to what I am working on. I've found it works best to go without my glasses and get up close. Finally, I have to manipulate items, mostly with one poorly coordinated hand. Thus, even simple "five-minute" jobs require an hour.

The inability to fix things may not seem like a big deal to many, but for me as a formerly avid do-it-yourselfer, it is extremely frustrating.

Finances

I am lucky. Many disabled people have significant worries about money. I do not. I have not had to handle any bills or insurance matters, just focus on recovery.

Credit my wife for this blessing. She has always handled the finances in our marriage. She has an MBA, though she doesn't use it anymore professionally. Our insurance is covered by her job as a teacher. Before the accident, I focused on earning money, then handed it to her. Since being hurt, she has done everything.

One large point in our favor is that before I was injured, we always lived very comfortably but not up to the level our income allowed. I lived like I hoped to retire early, whether or not I actually would do so. (Careful what you wish for.) Though our income has been dramatically reduced now, we have seen only modest changes in lifestyle. Combined with the divestment of many things, our prior savings mean we are in good shape financially. I get a nice disability income stream, and my living expenses are minimal (save a few medical things) since I cannot do all the hobbies I used to do.

I hope I don't sound like I'm bragging. If anything, this situation points out the truism of the old adage "you can't take it with you." Though I never felt like I sacrificed to save, I can't enjoy many of the fruits of my career.

Other Medical Issues

As we all get older (I'm in my late fifties now), health issues crop up. I have been fortunate so far to have only minor items.

I had a small skin cancer removed. The biopsy said it was a basal cell carcinoma, a non-serious type of cancer. Since I have always been fair and burn relatively easily, I have regular checkups with a dermatologist now.

I encountered BPH (benign prostatic hyperplasia) a few years back. Getting up several times each night to use the bathroom with a wheelchair is not fun. I keep the condition in check now with daily medication.

Speaking of less than enjoyable experiences, I have more frequent colonoscopies than most people, due to family history. Again, the wheelchair adds to the challenge of these tests.

Getting sick hits me very hard. Even a minor head cold

can have a big impact on my breathing and balance. For this reason, I make sure to get a flu shot each year.

Maybe this is a good place to share that swallowing pills needs extra focus. I can "lose" a pill in my mouth or throat since so much is numb. I don't really lose the medication since it is somewhere in my body, but having a bitter pill dissolve in some unknown location where I can taste it is not pleasant.

On the bright side, the numbness in my mouth on the right side makes some dental procedures proceed with less discomfort. I still take a local anesthetic just in case, but I am already numb.

Pets

We are cat people. Both my wife and I had a cat when we got married, and we've had several felines since. I have nothing against dogs and have had them at other times in my life. A cat simply proves easier to care for. Before the accident, I felt too busy to give a dog its proper attention. After I was hurt, I couldn't help much, so continuing with cats made an easy choice.

At the time I was injured, we had a single cat, a white rag-doll by the name of Schubert (named by my stepson after the composer). A woman from work took him in while I was in the hospital and rehab centers. Though we'd not had a formerly close relationship, Schubert basically adopted me when we both returned home. He would pad along ahead of me, looking back to ensure I was OK, when I used a rollator in the house. He often slept on my wheelchair when I was not sitting in it. He would lie on my chest on the sofa when

I took a nap. When I rolled my chair outside to get some sun, he would come out with me and, remarkably, come back in the house with me afterward.

Schubert finally passed away after several years. He had reached an age where it was not a shock. I felt relief that he had gone first. After their husbands died, both my mother and her sister were repeatedly attacked by their cats, and the cats had to be euthanized. I didn't want that to happen to Schubert if something took me.

We now have a pair of young cats, adopted from a shelter. They are not brothers but act that way. They haven't adopted me the way Schubert did, but over time (and since I am the one most at home) have grown closer. As I write this on the couch, one is sleeping in my vacant wheelchair.

Sex

Without going into details, yes, I can still have sex. It may not be the same or as frequent as before the accident, but my wife and I continue to share intimacy. I will not say anything further since doing so would violate our privacy.

Insects

I would never have guessed that biting insects would be a different experience after my accident, but they are. I have never liked bugs. One of the things I used to like best about hiking in the fall and winter is that I would not have to contend with flying insects.

At first blush, the numbness I feel would seem to be a blessing when it comes to insects. On the contrary, it is a curse. I can't feel insects when they alight or bite on a numb section of my body. They are free to dine without bother. I am not only defenseless but oblivious. Though the itching associated with the bites later is subdued, I eventually still feel it.

Another piece is that I can't hear bugs. I have actually had on a couple occasions a bite in my right ear canal without knowing it. I only figure it out later when I find blood when cleaning that ear.

Cleaning

If I were a fantasy character, I might be called the Bringer of Filth due to the dirt I track in on my wheelchair wheels. Having an outdoor chair helps, but it's mostly a seasonal issue. Though I rarely go out in truly foul weather, winter is difficult due to the sand and salt applied everywhere around here.

The big culprit seems to be the garage floor. I take my indoor chair into the garage to get into the car, but in the winter the floor has water and sand/salt that has come off the car. We wipe off my wheels when I go back inside, though it is not simple. My wife encourages me to get non-treaded wheelchair tires to make it easier to wipe them clean.

Entertaining

The preparation for entertaining at home is usually not a problem. Since I like to work in the kitchen, much of the baking usually falls to me. The cooking gets handled by my wife. Setting the table usually falls to my wife. This process hasn't changed dramatically from before my accident except I do more baking, less cooking now.

What has changed is that I can't do much except stay out of the way during the event itself. My wife has to do all the serving. Even worse, it is hard for me to chat with guests since I have trouble hearing them and they have (unsurprising) difficulty understanding my fractured speech. I sometimes catch a few words and can offer an intelligent comment, but most of the time I sit silently. Fortunately, my wife is a bright and skilled conversationalist.

Cleanup is another piece that falls to my wife. Again, it's mostly best if I just stay out of the way.

Hotels

When traveling, it is often simplest to stay in hotels if we have to stay overnight. Most private homes do not have the resources needed to accommodate a disabled person. Thanks to the ADA, nearly all hotels can manage a person in a wheelchair.

I've already written about carpeting and how it impairs what mobility I have. Most hotels use a thick-pile carpet so my movement is extremely limited.

Just because hotels comply with ADA regulations does not mean they are alike. Though all are usable, some shine brighter than others. A key area, of course, is in the bathroom. Grab rails are typical, but other features can vary. A lot. I won't get into the nuances of bathroom design since each person may have very different needs and preferences, but I will say that all disabled people should expect things to vary and to have to adapt. That's part of the travel experience, even if you're not injured.

Chapter 14

Coronavirus

I am probably one of the few people in the world whose appearance improves with a mask.

I always try to find a positive take. That habit is part of what helps me cope.

When I began to write this chapter, I didn't have that much to write about and wondered why I would devote a whole chapter to the subject of coronavirus. At that point, the pandemic hadn't changed my life much. I stopped going to PT and stepped up my exercise on my own for a while, but I rarely went out otherwise, so even the depths of a lockdown didn't affect my life much. Still, we were seeing only the first wave, so perhaps the impact on me would come later.

I was unsure—as were many of us—whether the disease would hit me severely if I got infected. I exercised and ate well and didn't have the sort of predisposing health conditions such that were usually discussed. On the other hand, my breathing remains slightly sketchy, and my ability to swallow continues to be compromised. I didn't want to burden the hospital or feel sick. As I expressed at the time, I felt I had used my lifetime quota of hours in an ICU, on a ventilator, and being intubated, so I wanted to leave that "fun" to others.

That's all a nice way of saying that the idea of going back to the ICU and intubation unnerved me. I like to think that I would survive the experience of assisted breathing and other life-saving measures if I needed them again, but I don't know if I have the strength anymore.

In addition, I didn't know how a case of Covid-19 would leave me. Of course, I could end up dead, though I'm not sure that would be the worst available outcome. Perhaps the virus would cause me to revert to tube feeding or be stuck in an institution with who knows what impairments. Or perhaps I would make a full recovery as so many did.

As a practical matter, lockdown did not hinder me much. I could still go cycling with my wife, continue to bake (although some ingredients ran short), and keep up my writing. Pandemics have often resulted in great works of literature. I didn't expect much since I was minimally affected.

Today, I am fully vaccinated, having never contracted Covid-19. I got the boosters when I became eligible. Life in Hanover is returning to normal, though variants rage. I still wear a mask as required at PT and elsewhere, but this is only a minor inconvenience.

In retrospect, I conclude that Covid-19 has had an impact on me, psychologically at least. While from the outside looking in, nothing much happened, what could have happened unsettled me in a way that wouldn't have occurred without my accident.

Chapter 15

Closing

A m I better off mood-wise than when I took that test shortly before I was hurt?

Am I still as unhappy as I once was? Was I just whining then? After all I have been through and have given up, the answer might seem obvious.

This book is a summary of my life as it has evolved. The quick conclusion would be that I can still do a lot, just very slowly and purposefully. And I get fatigued really fast.

I know a few people with brain injuries would not trade their life now for one without a TBI. I am not one of them. Yes, I am doing pretty well. I credit my family, my medical team, and dumb luck for making it this far. I have been the beneficiary of having good insurance coverage and plenty of savings. I have done what I can to move ahead in my diminished state, but I would have done something, maybe something great, if I hadn't been injured. Who knows. Conversely, maybe things were about to come crashing down if I hadn't been hurt. I was in danger, and this incident jerked me back from the edge.

I am not a fan of hypotheticals. Guessing what life would be like without a skull fracture doesn't help me. I do what I can with the reality that presents itself. Wishing things were different will not change the circumstances.

That said regarding the past, I can make some educated guesses about the future. I do not expect to recover further. While a miracle could always happen, it doesn't seem likely. I am probably at the peak of my abilities right now and hope to stay there as long as I can. I once told a therapist that one must strive to move forward or else one is automatically slipping back.

I will pass someday as all of us must do. Heart disease does not run in my family. That fact plus the constant aerobic work I do at PT and on the trike help me not to fear a heart problem. Cancer does, however, run in my family, so that area is a legitimate concern. As noted previously, I have had a small skin cancer already. Another possibility for me is some sort of degenerative neural disease. I certainly have less margin for losing brain tissue than an uninjured person.

Between exercise, working my brain, and regular medical care, I feel as well prepared for an uncertain future as I can be. I know nothing is assured and that a wide range of eventualities are possible. I will try to stay as independent as I can for as long as I can. None of us can ask for more.

One of the tragic things about being disabled is that I already look back on the years leading up to the accident as my glory days, professionally and personally. I suppose this is better than folks who peak in their teens or early twenties, but it still bothers me. I continue to try to create memorable times now, yet it is difficult.

Some people in my position might become cocky. The question would be: How much worse could it get? Rather, I tend toward the opposite. I know that so many of my present abilities hang by a slender thread. Any additional reduction in my physical or mental capacity could easily wreck what I have right now. I suppose this fact is no different than most able-bodied people. I guess I just have a heightened awareness, or perhaps less margin.

I recommend that one takes on whatever the struggle— be it a challenging job or disability—with a serious commitment without taking oneself too seriously. I try to live that way. For instance, a large part of my face remains numb. I say that some people pay a lot of money for Botox injections to achieve the same thing. Similarly, other folks go to great lengths to reside near the ocean where they can hear the surf. The loud rhythm of my pulse in my right ear approximates this sound and is always present.

I am sorry for the adverse impact of my injuries on others, especially my wife. This life is not what she signed up for. To her credit, she hasn't hesitated to support me. I do not look forward to the day when we will have been married longer with me hurt than prior to the accident.

As to a question that arises since I have become disabled: Am I a burden? First, I'll state that I think we (able-bodied and disabled alike) are all burdens. We all impose a cost by our existence. The question is really of burden to whom and whether our value generated offsets the cost in some way. Environmentally speaking, I'm arguably less a burden now than before my accident. Sure, I still eat and require climate control, among other things, yet I no longer drive a car, fly so readily, or use a powerboat. As for societal burden, I would argue that my status is largely a neutral factor, as I consume modest services yet provide employment to those that assist me.

I know I definitely am an increased burden to my family, but thus far everyone seems more than happy with having me around, so I guess it's a minor, or at least manageable, burden in their eyes.

So, returning to the question: How happy am I now? The answer might surprise some. Despite all of the challenges, I feel like I'm at least as happy as I used to be. Or maybe *contented* is a better word. Clearly, I'm different today, but not every change has been negative. I have physical challenges to deal with but also am far less stressed. I have less I can do but can address things I *can* do with more attention to detail. If I was looking for new heights to scale, I have no shortage now.

Psychological studies report that there seems to be a mood setpoint for each person, so that outside effects matter little to their intrinsic happiness. I seem to be a case study.

Early on I consciously decided to not be the depressed individual who feels sorry for himself. People will feel bad for you for only so long. No one wants to be around a pitiful figure all the time, including me. To avoid being isolated, I try to be positive. The reader is left to judge whether I have been successful in that pursuit.

Acknowledgments

I thank my coach, Deb Heimann, and everyone at Rootstock for helping me along this writing adventure. The staff at Creare made my engineering career very special.

I thank the first responders who dragged me out of the woods and the staff who stabilized me in the hospital in the Northeast Kingdom of Vermont. I am grateful for the care I received at Dartmouth-Hitchcock Medical Center, Spaulding Rehabilitation Hospital, and the Crotched Mountain head injury unit. My outpatient services when I got home were at DHMC, Alice Peck Day Memorial Hospital, Concord Hospital, and Cioffredi's Institute for Human Performance.

I thank my stepchildren, Nina and Jared, as well as the extended family on my wife's side for supporting me and their mother. I am also extremely grateful to my son, Jason, for his steadfast love and support, including frequent football discussions. I thank his mother, Libby, as well for making this process as easy as she could. I appreciate the continuing support of my high school and cycling buddies, Kurt and Nick. My brother, Mike, and his family have been very accommodating, especially on travel. Finally, I can't say thanks enough to my wife, Mary, for her love, care, and support in what has profoundly impacted her life as well.

About the Author

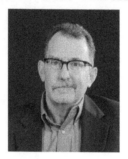

A native of Wisconsin, Jim Barry graduated from the University of Wisconsin-Madison with a PhD in nuclear engineering and engineering physics. He embarked on a three-decade career in research and development, rising to become president of one of the top firms in the country. His technical range was broad, including two-phase flow and heat transfer, aerosol dynamics, medical device design, chemical/biological protection, and computational fluid dynamics. He coauthored a number of technical papers and holds multiple patents. That career was cut short when he suffered a skull fracture and ensuing cerebral hemorrhage in a mountain biking crash (yes, he was wearing a helmet) that left him with limited mobility and limited verbal communication. He lives with his wife in New Hampshire.

More Nonfiction from Rootstock Publishing:

Also publishing fiction, poetry, and children's literature. Visit our website www.rootstockpublishing.com to learn more.

9 781578 691234